POSTPARTUM DIET BOOK FOR NEW MOMS

"Empowering New Moms: A Holistic Guide to Thrive in the Postpartum Odyssey"

Sharon D. Sletten

TABLE OF CONTENTS

Introduction

As you cradle your newborn baby for the very first time, an overwhelming wave of emotions floods over you. Joy, excitement, love - but also nervousness and doubt. Your world has changed in an instant and now a tiny human depends on you for everything.

In those first few hazy weeks of feedings, diaper changes and sporadic sleep, it's all too easy to put yourself and your needs last. But nourishing your body with a healthy postpartum diet is crucial during this transitional time. Proper nutrition helps boost recovery, energy, mood and milk supply - fueling you to be the best mother possible.

This book is here to take your hand and guide you through the murky waters of figuring out your own nutritional postpartum needs. Consider it your life raft, packed full of practical advice to simplify and demystify the what, when, why and how of eating well after giving birth. Expert wisdom distilled down into easily digestible nuggets.

Inside these pages you'll discover exactly which nutrients new moms require most, which foods deliver them, meal planning strategies and hacks for quick prep and one-handed eating when the baby demands to be held 24/7. You'll find support for navigating challenges like loss of appetite, gastrointestinal issues, postpartum weight loss, food sensitivities and allergies. Plus tips for wholesome nutrition on a budget and when time is at a premium.

With the help of this book, self-care won't need to be yet another item on your endless to-do list. You'll gain confidence in your ability to nourish both your baby and your body, gracefully balancing the needs of your new expanded family. Regain vibrancy, feel like yourself again - heal from within and glow from the outside.

The transformation begins one bite at a time! Now let's get you properly fueled...

<u>Welcome to the Postpartum Journey</u>
Congratulations mama! However long you laboured and however intense your delivery, your baby has arrived safely into this world. As you hold that precious new life in your arms perhaps you feel elated, awestruck, relieved or completely drained – or some complex cocktail of all of those emotions.

Whatever thoughts race through your exhausted mind in these first hours and days postpartum, your body has some major adjusting ahead after 10 months of growing and nurturing another human. The journey doesn't stop just because birth is behind you. Your body must navigate profound metabolic, hormonal and physical shifts to move from a pregnancy state to supporting a breastfeeding mother.

This transition is a marathon event, not a sprint. Be gently patient with yourself as changes unfold slowly over 6-8 weeks' time or longer. Making smart nutritional choices will fuel and speed the adjustment. The postpartum period shapes future health so high quality fuel matters! That's where this book comes in as your nutritional road map for recovering well and thriving after childbirth.

Starting Off Well-Nourished

Every new mom deserves proper nourishment while her body stitches itself back together after the rigours of labour, delivery and any necessary procedures. Stocking up on the right foods beforehand means you won't need to stress about nutrition when you'd rather just rest, bond and care for a baby in those first tender days.

Plan easy meals for your hospital bag like protein bars, nuts, fruits and veggies you can nibble one-handed. Have your partner prepare nourishing snacks and dishes to await you when you get home. Soups, stews, fresh produce, eggs, yoghurt, oats and more whole foods help the healing journey. Stay hydrated with water and avoid overly salty foods causing fluid retention or constipation.

Key Nutrients for Recovery

Each aspect of your postpartum recovery places high demands upon your nutrient stores so optimising your intake both speeds healing and safeguards your future health. Let's explore key vitamins, minerals and macronutrients enabling your body's many transformations.

Protein – Building Blocks for Healing Tissues

From the first moments postpartum, mama's body enters rebuild and repair mode. Birthing a baby leaves vaginal tears, episiotomies, haemorrhoids, sore muscles and other tissue trauma needing mending back to wholeness. Your blood volume drops profoundly from fluid shifts so increasing hematopoiesis depends upon abundant protein for crafting fresh red blood cells and clotting factors. Milk protein production also taps maternal reserves.

Aim for at least 80-100g of high-quality protein sources like eggs, poultry, fish/seafood, Greek yoghurt, cottage cheese, nuts/seeds, beans/legumes and lean red meat if your iron stores need replenishing after blood loss. Dietary protein also promotes the liver's detoxification enzymes aiding natural postpartum cleansing processes.

Iron – Oxygen Delivery to Revitalise Fatigued Cells

Iron enables haemoglobin molecules inside red blood cells to carry oxygen, fueling the entire body's healing energy needs. But blood loss from delivery, prolonged nursing sessions and night sweats all drain iron stores. Postpartum anaemia leaves over 70% of new moms low on this precious mineral, causing exhaustion, slowed recovery, susceptibility to postpartum infections and challenges like depression.

Red meat provides the most bioavailable iron but also seeks out poultry, eggs, legumes, spinach and iron-fortified cereals/breads. Pair iron-rich foods with vitamin C from citrus, peppers, kiwi and berries which improves iron absorption up to six-fold! Avoid excess calcium and coffee caffeine which hinder iron uptake.

Vitamin C – Immune Support & Wound Healing

Staving off postpartum infections to keep mama and baby healthy ranks among your top recovery goals. Vitamin C builds resilient immune defences and this antioxidant also manufactures fresh collagen for sealing up damaged tissues. A Swiss study found postpartum women require 100-200 mg daily, over twice normal levels, to optimise convalescence based on vitamin C blood concentration decline after delivery.

Fruits and vegetables brimming with vitamin C like citrus, mango, papaya, red bell peppers, broccoli, tomatoes and dark leafy greens help wounds mend quickly while bolstering immunity. Enjoy raw whenever possible since cooking saps up to 50% of vitamin C content from produce. Supplement if dietary sources fall short.

Omega-3s – Hormonal Harmony & Neurological Development

From modulating inflammation and mood to forming healthy neurons in a baby's rapidly developing brain, omega-3 fatty acids offer wide-ranging postpartum and lactation support. These special fats integrating into cell membranes help normalise surging post-birth hormones like prolactin and oxytocin. Research reveals new moms with adequate omega-3 status have a lower likelihood of postpartum depression, faster recovery and reduced arthritis flare risk.

Seafood, especially cold water fatty fish like salmon, mackerel and sardines, provides eicosapentaenoic acid (EPA) and docosahexaenoic acid (DHA). Grass-fed meat, eggs, walnuts and flaxseeds deliver plant-derived ALA converted somewhat inefficiently to EPA and DHA so vegetarian moms should supplement. Most prenatals provide DHA but levels often prove insufficient for nursing mothers.

Probiotics & Prebiotics – Gut & Vaginal Microbiome Recovery

From wrenching hormones to antibiotic exposures, the entire postpartum period intensely disturbs delicate microbial ecologies. Profound gut flora shifts make many new mamas miserable with bloating, gas, abdominal pain and erratic bowel patterns. Perineal microbes face chaotic upheaval after physical birth trauma coupled with pad use and poor hygiene potentially causing infections.

Supporting vulnerable microbiomes with "good" bugs and their nourishing prebiotic fibres jumpstarts recovery for both digestion and feminine health. Consume plenty of fermented foods like unsweetened yoghourt, kefir, kimchi, kombucha, sauerkraut and pickled veggies. Seek out probiotic supplements explicitly balancing postpartum gut flora strains shown to dial down inflammation and reinforce immunity.

Prebiotic fibres that act as fertilisers for healthy microbes come from onion, garlic, asparagus, Jerusalem artichokes, dandelion greens, chicory root and especially breastmilk! Yes, encouraging frequent nursing inoculates babies with your custom probiotics. Win-win nutrition in action.

Key Micronutrients – Multivitamin Insurance

Healing tissues and producing breast milk to nourish a newborn become incredibly micronutrient-intensive for postpartum mothers. Demand often outpaces dietary sources for critical agents like vitamin D regulating inflammatory balance, B vitamins energising metabolism, zinc assisting immunity and wound closure, magnesium easing hormonal mood swings and calcium/phosphorus constructing bone and teeth.

Rather than tracking dozens of individual micrograms and milligrams, most mammals benefit from a high-quality, third-party verified postnatal multivitamin delivering sufficient quantities until intake stabilises. If food restrictions or aversions make achieving minimums unlikely for vulnerable vitamins like B12, folate, zinc or vitamin C, please supplement accordingly. Setting yourself up for success with optimal nutrition now echoes through generations.

<u>Importance of a Balanced Postpartum Diet</u>
After nearly a year of shifting priorities and major bodily changes preparing for motherhood culminates in birth, new mamas rightfully feel eager to reclaim their pre-baby bodies. But patience proves paramount during the postpartum period spanning at least six weeks and ideally three months or longer. This transitional healing phase shapes your health and wellbeing for years so approach self-care gently but diligently.

Now more than ever, a balanced diet provides the essential ingredients for supporting this total body overhaul. Nutrients fuel every major system aiding postpartum recovery from cellular repair to milk supply. They balance rollercoaster hormones, temper inflammatory forces, lift energy, brighten mood and empower immunity. Alongside rest, balanced nutrition lays the strongest foundation for gracefully adapting to life with your new baby.

Postpartum Nutritional Needs

During pregnancy your body's nutrient demands increased to support the developing baby. So what changes after birth? Requirements for most vitamins and minerals remain significantly elevated to promote healing, milk production and sustain this period of high physical stress. Your postpartum diet should emphasise whole, minimally processed foods delivering enough high-quality macronutrients, micronutrients and antioxidants for recovering well.

Calories – Finding a New Normal

Calorie needs naturally shift as pregnancy's third trimester energy surplus converts into lactation's increased demands, just as bump gives way to baby in arms. Most women require around 400 extra calories for breastfeeding over pre-pregnancy intake, equivalent to 2 servings of grain, protein or dairy. Listen to internal hunger and fullness cues without forcing excess food or deliberately limiting calories.

Postpartum weight changes vary widely - losing baby weight rapidly doesn't indicate health. Pace yourself, especially if breastfeeding, because extreme energy deficits can tank milk supply and retard healing. Emphasise wholesome sources providing enough protein first before counting calories. Trust your body knows how to find its new normal in time.

Macronutrients – High Quality Fuel Matters

Carbohydrates offer quick fuel to power healing tissues but focus on less refined, higher fibre sources like whole grains, starchy vegetables, fruits and legumes instead of simple sweets. Avoid driving blood sugar spikes and inflammation with excessive sugary treats. Each meal should contain moderate protein for repairing muscles, skin, organs plus milk components if breastfeeding. Healthy fats enhance hormone balance, inflammation modulation and satisfy appetite. Obtained from oily fish, nuts, seeds, avocados, extra virgin olive oil and full-fat dairy.

Micronutrients – Insurance for Recovery

Vitamins and minerals enable countless essential reactions supporting convalescence. Postpartum nutrient depletion causes symptoms slowing progress like fatigue, impaired immunity, low mood, poor wound healing, headaches, GI issues and more. Avoid deficits in key supporters like iron, magnesium, B vitamins, zinc, vitamin C and omega-3s through a colourful balanced diet. Consider filling any gaps with a multi designed specifically to meet elevated needs.

Water – Hydration Helps Healing

Rehydrating after fluid losses from delivery, sweating, bleeding and breastfeeding proves pivotal for postpartum recovery. Drink to thirst focusing on water as well as herbal teas, broths and milk. Signs of lingering dehydration like constipation, darkened urine, fatigue or headaches signal a need for more fluids. Stay well hydrated and notice if dietary choices like excess caffeine, sugar or salt counteract hydration.

Gut Support for Nutrient Absorption

Postpartum digestive function often lags thanks to shifting hormones, antibiotics exposure during labour and physical after-effects like haemorrhoids. Healthy gut flora and gentle motility both enable optimal utilisation of all the balanced nutrition you provide. Consume fermented foods, high fibre plant foods and probiotic supplements to repopulate digestive health. Stay active, attempt elimination daily and avoid straining.

Nourishing the Future

Your postpartum nutrition sets the stage for lifelong health through lactation nutrition benefiting infants and by balancing accumulation of inflammatory visceral fat shown to raise future chronic disease risk. This ephemeral window shapes not just recovery and return to pre-baby shape but more critically long term wellbeing for both mother and child. Prioritise self-care knowing your choices now ripple through generations as your baby grows healthy and strong.

Eating for Balance, Harmony and Healing
Your individual postpartum nutrition plan must nourish a recovering body while reflecting current needs and capabilities. What does balanced eating mean for a sleep-deprived mama struggling with a fussy

newborn around the clock? Or dealing with food aversions, nausea or appetite changes? Be adaptable and resilient without rigid rules. Make each bite count without striving for perfection.

Focus first on emphasising minimally processed sources of essential proteins, healthful fats and complex carbohydrates to fuel rapid healing. Then expand dietary variety and balance each time the baby permits. Customise your diet to serve this temporary but pivotal phase best. Seek balance over the long haul rather than expecting each meal to meet all needs. Extend grace knowing this too shall pass as you both adjust.

Every new mom wants to sprint through postpartum changes straight into her old jeans but respect the distance of this ultra-marathon. You must walk – slowly, deliberately, lovingly – each step of the way. Nourish body and soul along this precious journey, trusting your body to reveal in time a new balance both similar yet forever changed from your pre-baby days. Keep perspective on what matters most, just like your perfect new baby.

Navigating the Challenges of Postpartum Nutrition

The rapid physical and emotional changes ushered in by childbirth present new mamas with ample challenges during the postpartum period. Shifting priorities coupled with sheer exhaustion from erratic sleep easily distract from self-care. But paying attention to signals from your body proves pivotal now for both recovering well and avoiding long-lasting ramifications of nutritional stress that manifest years later.

You need proper fuel and hydration to heal, balance tempestuous hormones, produce plenty of milk for baby, lift energy, brighten mood and empower immunity. Easier said than done while adjusting to an infant dictating your entire schedule! By understanding common nutritional hurdles after giving birth, you can establish resilience and adaptability to meet this temporary but significant physiological transition. Here's how to navigate the choppy waters of postpartum nutrition.

Diminished Appetite

In the wake of labour's intense physical expenditure, some mamas emerge ravenously hungry, rapidly devouring meals. But more often extreme fatigue coupled with digestive slowdown leaves little desire for food despite heightened needs. Between latch issues, sore nipples, engorgement and cluster feeding, the demands of breastfeeding also curb appetite drive.

Nausea, abdominal bloating, hemorrhoid discomfort and hormonal fluctuations further erode appetite for many women through early postpartum. Prioritising rest and asking for help with baby care supports the body conserving energy for recovery instead of digestion. Don't force feed but do emphasise snacks and smaller balanced meals every few hours. The urge to graze returns soon, especially as milk production escalates hunger!

Food Aversions & Cravings

Thanks to wildly fluctuating oestrogen, progesterone and cortisol influencing taste receptors and brain chemistry, your postpartum food preferences may bear little resemblance to pre-pregnancy cravings! Changing odour sensitivities, often amplified by nausea or fatigue, introduce new aversions to formerly favourite flavours. Sudden distaste for meat, eggs, spices or other nourishing proteins leaves minimal appeal for crucial building blocks.

Simultaneously cravings often emerge for quick carbohydrate fixes like pasta, bread, sugar cereal and sweets rather than high fibre whole grains providing steady energy. Attuning to signals from your body's inner wisdom helps guide intuitive eating to overcome rollercoaster appetite changes. Getting enough nutrition may require creative approaches for this temporary phase.

Gastrointestinal Woes

From the earliest post-delivery hours, digestive function faces downhill challenges between pain meds, antibiotic exposures, slowed motility from bed rest and elevated stress hormones. Prolonged pressure during labour and delivery can trigger hemorrhoid inflammation further aggravating elimination. Constipation results, often paired with stranded gas and bloating causing discomfort.

Some women also develop postpartum diarrhoea, typically from a major shift in gut microbes after antibiotics or from hormonal influence on intestinal secretions. Finding gentle relief without straining proves important although modifying diet can also help by increasing hydration and fibre while avoiding dairy, fat or irritating foods if diarrhoea results. Probiotics, magnesium and omega-3s ease GI upset.

Extreme Fatigue

You expect sleep deprivation with a newborn but postpartum hormonal shifts severely worsen fatigue for at least the first month and often longer. Night sweats, restless legs, vivid dreams and waking to feed the baby prevent restorative rest. Postnatal nutrient depletion, blood volume loss, inflammation and pain all deepen exhaustion too. Light exercise boosts energy somewhat but cordoning off naps remains essential.

Rather than fighting fatigue, flow with your body's signals to slow down and sleep whenever possible. Lowering other demands and obligations allows conservation of energy for recovery. Identify quick, easy-to-assemble snacks and meals for those intervals when baby naps. Select more cold foods requiring little prep like smoothies, no-cook oats, salads, cottage cheese.

Mood Instability

Maternal mood gets thrown completely off kilter after childbirth thanks to radical hormone shifts. Postpartum depression receives due attention but a spectrum of anxiety, irritability, anger, sadness and other symptoms plague around 80% of new moms for weeks until hormones re-equilibrate. Imbalanced brain chemistry coupled with fatigue and feeling overwhelmed predispose women to mood disorders.

Regulate emotional surges first through self-care basics like sleeping enough, resetting expectations about "doing it all" and lowering other stressors. Counselling, meditation, sage smudging, prayer and journaling also help. Dietary efforts emphasising protein, healthy fats and colourful plant foods provide building blocks for neurotransmitters influencing mood.

Managing Postpartum Weight Loss

Media fixates on celebrity post-baby body reveals as though snapping right back to pre-pregnancy form after delivering new life reflects health. In reality, postpartum metabolism and body composition shifts need gentle care and patience. Expecting substantial weight loss while breastfeeding works against milk supply and recovery. But some new mamas still push overly hard for fast results either from anxiety or social messaging.

Composition changes like increased body fat support lactation by steadying energy supply. Less visceral and liver fat benefits future maternal health. Relax about the scale and avoid actively dieting, calorie counting or eliminating food groups unless medically advised. Instead emphasise whole, nutritious sources that leave you feeling satisfied. Weight finds its set point later, after weaning.

The key to sailing smoothly through the stormy seas of postpartum nutrition involves flexibility, self-compassion and adaptation guided by functional signals from your body. What does a baby need nutritionally right now? What supports healing best today? What foods bring comfort versus distress? rather than following rigid rules. Get creative, stay patient with changes and trust your inner wisdom. This too shall pass!

Chapter 1: Nutritional Needs During the Postpartum Period

Pregnancy nutrition serves to nourish all the amazing bodily preparation and transitions unfolding to bring your miracle baby into the world. But the needs shift yet again during the postpartum period as labour and the enormous feat of delivery exert intense demands on mama's depleted reserves. Recovery processes accelerate regeneration while many women simultaneously summon the energy for round the clock infant care and milk production.

The postpartum rollercoaster ride requires key nutrients in elevated amounts to keep fatigue, infection risk, poor wound healing, thyroid dysfunction, mood swings and suboptimal lactation at bay. Achieving nutritional sufficiency from diet alone proves difficult, even under ideal conditions. Restoring nutrient stores serves your own wellness interests as well as the baby's lifelong health imprinted by these precious early months.

Macronutrients – Protein, Healthy Fats & Carbohydrates

You might expect the composition of breastmilk to perfectly reflect the proportions of macronutrients needed for postpartum recovery. In fact, breast milk contains far more lactose (a carbohydrate) for nourishing rapid infant brain development than the extra protein and fat maternal tissues need to regenerate from delivery trauma. Postpartum priorities shift from purely baby-centric nourishment toward more maternal centred healing wisdom.

Replenish with ample protein foods like eggs, poultry, fatty fish, Greek yoghurt, cottage cheese, nut butters, beans and lentils. Your body breaks down those amino acids into materials for repairing uterine tissues, vaginal tears, haemorrhoids, skin elasticity, strained muscles, depleted blood volume and more. Protein also prevents excessive breast milk volume loss when calories drop.

Healthy fats calm inflammation, balance rollercoaster hormones, support mood and satisfy appetite between meals. Emphasise omega-3 rich sources like salmon, sardines, walnuts and flax. Other nourishing fats come from olive oil, coconut, avocados, and full-fat dairy. Complex carbohydrates provide sustaining energy for all the healing action without spiking blood sugar. Seek fibre-rich whole grains, starchy vegetables, fruits and legumes.

Key Micronutrients – Vitamins, Minerals & Antioxidants

Delivering life force to another human leaves a new mom depleted across micronutrients – no matter how exemplary her pregnancy diet! Blood volume and iron loss may trigger anaemia while immune resilience depends upon zinc, vitamin C and vitamin D. Neurotransmitters lifting mood and energy require B vitamins, magnesium and omega-3s. Milk supply and recovering hormones run on calcium, iodine and vitamin A.

Eating a spectrum of nutrient dense whole foods helps prevent postnatal deficits but almost all women benefit from insurance in the form of a comprehensive multivitamin delivering at least the recommended daily dose for pregnancy and ideally even higher levels for key postpartum nutrients. Breastfeeding mothers especially need extra nutrients that directly translate into optimal nutrition for the baby through milk's components.

Water & Electrolytes

Meeting amplified fluid needs often proves overlooked after delivery yet critical for replenishing blood volume, enabling milk production, supporting digestion and flushing inflammation and toxins. Aim for at least 3 litres of total fluid daily from water, herbal tea, broths and milk. Coconut water offers efficacious electrolyte support. Signs of lingering dehydration like fatigue, headache and dark urine signal drink more!

Probiotics & Prebiotics

Antibiotics exposure during labour, haemorrhoids discomfort, profound hormonal shifts and peri-delivery microflora changes leave many new mamas struggling with postpartum digestion ranging from constipation to diarrhoea plus gas and bloating. Supporting microbiome balance with daily probiotic supplements benefits gut health and motility while also preventing dysbiosis-related issues like mastitis or vaginal infections through the 6-8 week healing window and into sustained breastfeeding.

Prebiotic fibres from whole plant foods, nuts and seeds also feed friendly flora. Prioritising fermented items like unsweetened yoghurt, kefir, kombucha, kimchi and sauerkraut provide natural probiotics. Healthy digestion and immunity both depend upon balanced microflora so consume these daily.

Adapt as Needed

Postpartum nutritional needs remain elevated throughout lactation to fuel milk quality and support sprinkling in new baby-centric priorities amidst healing. But demands and capabilities change daily, even hourly! Adapt food choices to suit your current energy levels, appetite, aversions or cravings, digestive function, convenient options and how a baby feels about letting you set him/her down to snack!

What matters most involves emphasising whole food nourishment whenever possible, staying hydrated, getting some sunlight daily, taking a maternal-centric multivitamin and being gently forgiving with yourself when plans get toppled. Meet needs as best as circumstances allow while focusing on superfoods offering maximum nutritional bang for the bite. This too shall pass!

Impact of Breastfeeding on Dietary Requirements

Among the myriad changes new motherhood brings, establishing a breastfeeding relationship ranks among the most intimate and potentially challenging. Despite mom's best efforts, latch or supply issues arise more often than Instagram tales might imply! Navigating nursing difficulties while also recovering from delivery and baby's round-the-clock needs leaves little time for properly fueling your own body.

Yet meeting amplified nutritional needs now potently influences milk quality and quantity plus your capacity to meet mounting demands. Breastfeeding exerts substantial dietary impacts spanning calories required, optimal macro and micronutrients, hydration needs and even digestion. Understanding exactly how lactation shifts priorities and appetite provides the first step toward fueling this incredible but depleting process.

Calorie Needs - Breastfeeding Hunger!

Producing the approximately 25-35 oz of milk baby requires daily to thrive significantly boosts mama's calorie burn by at least 400 but often closer to 500 extra calories beyond pre-pregnancy needs. The energy for milk production comes first from mom's diet then from stored body fat if intake falls short. Weight drops rapidly for some women thanks to this built-in calorie deficit.

Yet deliberately limiting calories or actively "eating for two" by overconsuming both prove counterproductive for successfully breastfeeding. Survival hunger ruled by appetite and cravings offers the best nutrition guide. Listen for cues to eat frequently - every 2-4 hours. Emphasise varied whole foods delivering enough protein first before counting calories. Drink to thirst and snack despite any pressure to fast for weight loss.

Macronutrients: Protein, Fat and Carbohydrates

Protein provides amino acid building blocks to craft milk's bioactive compounds, antibodies and enzymes baby's growing body and mind requires. As needs for tissue repair from delivery wane, more dietary protein shuttles directly into milk. Low protein intake causes low milk volume yet excess protein also strains kidneys processing waste. Stick to recommended daily intake of at least 60-100 grams/day from eggs, poultry, fish, Greek yoghurt, nuts, beans, etc.

Healthy fats aid lactation through improving hormone signals, reducing inflammation and enhancing digestion. Omega-3s regulate milk fat composition while medium chain triglycerides in coconut oil boost supply. Seek salmon, nut butters, extra virgin olive oil, avocados. Quick burning carbs like fruits, whole grains and starchy vegetables offer the preferred fuel for milk production over protein or fat. Ideally timed intake prevents energy crashes.

Vitamins and Minerals

Manufacturing a whole other human's food supply from scratch every day for months or even years requires bountiful micronutrients! B vitamins activate energy cycles, vitamin C enables immune factors in milk and mineral electrolytes provide ingredients for optimal nutrient balance benefiting the baby. Replace depleted vitamin D for mood, bone health and battling inflammation - critical for nursing mothers.

Seek out vitamin and mineral replenishment from veggies, fruits, whole grains, beans, nuts, seeds and lean proteins. A prenatal vitamin extends insurance but the ideal choice for breastfeeding is a dedicated lactation multivitamin formulated with higher levels of key supporters like iodine for thyroid function, zinc for immunity and milk production plus extra calcium for your own bone health.

Hydration Needs Double

Making milk requires substantial maternal fluid reserves so daily needs jump while breastfeeding. Dehydration compromises supply rapidly but few mothers heed this red flag soon enough, attributing low output to other issues first. Drink frequently even without thirst to combat unavoidable losses from sweating, milk production and energy expenditure.

Fluids holding electrolytes prove most efficacious for electrolyte losses via milk like coconut water and diluted fruit juices. Otherwise emphasise ample pure water, herbal tea, broths and milk. Signs like dark urine, fatigue or headaches means more hydration urgently needed. Don't overlook this simplest requirement for bountiful milk and energy.

Gut Support for Nutrient Assimilation

You must absorb and assimilate all the balanced nutrition you carefully consume in order for quality breastmilk to result! But postpartum digestion still recovers from hormonal shifts plus antibiotics exposure during labour as pregnancy's progesterone relaxes its grip. Gut microbes face chaos after physical delivery changes. Gas, bloating and stool irregularities often linger for weeks or months.

Support microbiome balance by eating fermented foods like yoghurt, kefir and kimchi plus daily probiotic supplements. Increase plant fibre intake through fruits, veggies, beans and whole grains that act as prebiotics - food for friendly flora. Address new sensitivities if dairy, gluten, nuts or other formerly favourite foods now trigger digestive distress flaring inflammation and worsening fatigue. Heal the gut for increased energy liberation from all nourishing foods.

In the same way the baby thrives best with milk perfectly personalised rather than formula, meet YOUR unique nutritional needs in the postpartum period by listening closely and responding intuitively. Follow appetite guides, support digestion, hydrate almost excessively and emphasise a rainbow of whole foods delivering enough protein and healthy fats first before tracking calories. Trust your body's innate wisdom to signal exactly how to eat for abundant energy to nourish and heal you both!

<u>Addressing Common Nutrient Deficiencies</u>
The monumental feat of nurturing new life leaves a postpartum mama depleted, stressed and seriously nutritionally vulnerable. Demands to recover from delivery, adjust to parenting, produce ample milk, regulate unstable hormones and prevent infections all depend upon crucial vitamins, minerals, antioxidants, protein and healthy fats. Yet fatigue, nausea, losing muscle for milk amino acids, blood volume reductions and frequent use of antibiotics synergize to exhaust stores.

Alongside adequate catch-up sleep and self care, replacing missing nutrients offers a foundational strategy for restoring your body from cellular to emotional levels. Let's explore six of the most frequently developing postnatal and lactation nutrient gaps interfering with full wellness restoration so you can replenish effectively.

Iron - Restoring Oxygen Energy

Iron ranks as the most common nutritional deficiency after childbirth thanks to the double drain of blood volume loss during delivery followed by rapid use for restoring red blood cells plus feeding another human through breast milk.Postpartum anaemia leaves over 70% of mothers depleted, slowing recovery and physical capability while tanking mood, energy, immunity and thyroid function.

Replenishing iron requires deliberately seeking ample dietary sources like grass-fed red meat, organ meats like liver or heart, dark turkey meat, eggs and pumpkin seeds. Combine Vitamin C rich foods to enhance absorption yet avoid excess calcium or coffee that can limit uptake. Chat with your provider about the benefit/risk ratio of iron supplementation tailored to your needs.

Magnesium - Stress Resilience Mineral

This miracle mineral ranks nearly as abundant as iron with deficiencies after frequent use of antibiotics, blood or protein loss, or using stores faster than eating magnesium foods thanks to unchecked inflammation and stress. Results range from anxiety and insomnia to headaches, leg cramps, low energy, gut issues and more.

Pumpkin seeds hold excellent magnesium but leafy greens, nuts, whole grains, legumes, avocado, dark chocolate and fatty fish also contribute dietary magnesium. Absorption increased through vitamin D so sourced from the sun or supplements if needed. Consider 200-400 mg/day in supplemental form such as magnesium glycinate or citrate which the body absorbs and utilises well.

Vitamin D - Mood, Immunity and Inflammation Support

Few new moms get enough sun exposure for adequate cutaneous vitamin D synthesis thanks to new baby care duties relegating women indoors. Yet this pivotal nutrient makes hormones and neurotransmitters for balancing mood, enables immune cells and helps resolve postpartum inflammation. Depletion leaves women prone to depression, thyroid dysfunction, impaired healing, osteoporosis and upper respiratory infections.

Prioritise a short walk in midday sunlight but also consider an oral supplement delivering 2,000-4,000 IUs of D3 daily through winter months or year round if you live far from the equator. Vitamin D works synergistically with other fat soluble nutrients A, E and K2 so emphasise plenty of leafy greens and unprocessed plant oils like olive oil in cooking.

Probiotics - Microbiome Support

Healthy postpartum digestion depends upon balanced gut flora plus excellent motility. But labour antibiotics devastate beneficial bacteria leaving immune and detox pathways weakened. Pain meds, delivery mode changes and antibiotics passed via breast milk also disrupt infant flora. Lactation further depletes strains like bifidobacteria present in more than fifty times higher amounts in mom's milk than typical probiotics supply.

Bridge the gaps by eating probiotic rich fermented foods like miso, kimchi, kefir, kombucha, sauerkraut, pickled veggies and yoghurt. Additionally supplement with at least 30 billion CFUs daily from a multi-strain, shelf-stable probiotic. Target additional Bifidobacterium and Saccharomyces strains specialised to optimise mom and baby microbiomes. Sugar cravings and post meal fatigue signal imbalanced gut flora needing support.

Omega 3s - Hormonal Harmony

Intense hormonal shifts after delivering placenta combined with oestrogen influences on supply and prolactin for milk production involve delicate dance. Making ample DHA/EPA omega-3 fatty acids enables smooth signalling of receptors ensuring equilibrium not unhinged chaos. Always seek omega-3s from low toxin sources like sardines, wild caught salmon or algae oil over flax or other high omega-6 vegetable oils.

If not obtaining 2-3 grams daily from seafood, consider an algae oil supplement delivering at least 1000 mg combined DHA+EPA for mood stabilisation, blood sugar regulation and dialling down harmful postpartum inflammatory cascades. Add other sources like grass fed meat, walnuts or chia seeds to meet amplified needs of at least 1500 mg while breastfeeding.

Iodine – Thyroid Hormone and Brain Booster

Producing substantial calories in milk daily can drain iodine reserves rapidly given this mineral plays a starring role as essential constituent of key lactation hormones oxytocin, prolactin and thyroxine dictating supply. Iodine enables healthy thyroid functioning to balance energy, mood and metabolism - especially pivotal postpartum. And a baby's developing brain requires iodine all through pregnancy and nursing for optimal IQ boost.

Seaweed, seafood, eggs, strawberries and navy beans offer dietary iodine but amounts vary widely. A dedicated supplement containing 225-500 mcg of potassium iodide often fills gaps most efficacious for nursing mothers and babies unless you eat copious amounts of seaweed daily! This protects maternal thyroid health and baby's neurodevelopment.

While each woman's postpartum period unfolds uniquely, virtually all new mothers stand to gain strength, energy, confidence and a sense of calm from providing their body extra nutritional care including gentle supplementation to fill inevitable gaps. Establishing resilience now echoes through the coming months and years of raising your precious child. Healing from within lights your ability to shine bright guiding their journey through life!

Chapter 2: Building a Strong Foundation

The awe-inspiring yet exhausting path to new motherhood fundamentally transforms a woman's physiology and priorities in the space of a few short hours. As you embrace a tiny, perfect new life into your arms perhaps you alternatingly thrill with elation and shiver with doubt over providing for this helpless infant now 100% dependent on your care. Delivering a child leaves little time to focus on rebuilding your own depleted body. But self-care forms the cornerstone for thriving in your extended family.

Regaining resilience through excellent nutrition, ample rest and self-compassion shepherds you through the postpartum marathon. What you eat now not only fuels a gentle return to vibrancy but also potently shapes a baby's lifelong health through breastmilk's composition and epigenetic messaging. Building back better brightens the landscape for your little one to flourish.

Where do you start to construct a strong foundation?

Stock Your Healing Pantry

Before the baby makes their grand entrance, take time to shop for and prepare nourishing postpartum foods to keep hunger, headaches and low energy at bay. Stock your freezer, fridge and pantry with simple proteins, snacks you can eat one-handed, fresh fruits/veggies, nuts/seeds for snacking, quick baked goods like muffins and enough hydrating beverages so you needn't rush out shopping the first couple weeks.

Emphasise ingredients naturally boosting recovery: salmon, sardines and eggs for protein and omega-3s; bananas, avocado and cooked greens to avoid digestion taxing raw salads; probiotic yoghurts and kefir; citrus fruits, berries, tomatoes flooding your system with vitamin C and antioxidants; zinc-rich seeds and whole grains; magnesium restoring nuts and dark chocolate for mood; ginger, mint and chamomile tea to settle stomach; and broths delivering hydration alongside electrolytes and easily absorbed minerals.

Craft an Initial Meal Plan

Scheming out a few easy but nourishing recipes before late pregnancy fatigue sets in can offer new-mom-you salvation. Identify dishes you can assemble quickly or just throw in the crockpot like stews, chilis, bone broth soups and casseroles along with baked goods freezing well like muffins, lactation cookies and banana bread loaves. Stock pre-prepped healthy snacks like veggies with hummus, boiled eggs, cheese, fruit and mixed nuts.

Plan to rely on simple proteins, produce, healthy fats and complex carbs providing steady energy instead of sugar spikes and crashes leaving you ravenous. Whole food nourishment supports hormonal harmony, milk quality, mental clarity and avoidance of unhealthy postpartum weight loss pathways like excess cortisol. Diet diversity protects microbiomes and bolsters resilience so emphasises a vibrant, rainbow coloured foundation.

Support Nutrient Sufficiency

In the rush and exhaustion of new motherhood, perfectly balanced daily nutrition often slides down the priority list. But gently bridging common postnatal depletion supports mood balance, energy restoration, healing and infection prevention building momentum not deficits. Seek out high quality prenatal supplements delivering enough iron, magnesium, zinc and B vitamins alongside sufficient protein foods, omega-3s and probiotics.

Set yourself up for success by choosing minimally processed snacks, foods and beverages requiring little preparation yet providing maximum nutritional benefit. Stockpile frozen berries for smoothies, nuts to grab on the go, celery sticks and nut butter rather than highly refined packaged items. Structure promotes consistency so develop a few fallback easy meals relying on habitual ingredients from your healing pantry.

Move Gently, Rest Deeply

New mothers often push to rush through recovery, resume exercise too quickly and ignore pleading signals from their body for rest. But conserving your precious energy allows natural healing wisdom to work its magic. Gentle movement like walking, stretching or prenatal yoga supports circulation and reconnects you to your changing form without taxing depleted reserves.

Equally prioritise extended rest periods whenever possible. Let non-essential tasks slide to catch treasured naps and sleep longer overnight stretches by recruiting family support with meals and baby care. Say no to pressures pulling you from critically needed sleep fueling mood, milk supply and rebuilding strength. This too shall pass but right now your body beckons you to slow down.

Honour Your Authentic Needs

Every woman's postpartum experience unfolds uniquely according to delivery factors, infant temperament, her support network and background health status. Ditch rigid assumptions around "normal". Instead grow skills for attuning to your authentic needs through journaling, meditation or simply taking 5 deep belly breaths before reacting. What food or activities feel nourishing versus draining right now? How can you thoughtfully support your body's wisdom in the coming days?

Building resilient foundations for thriving in your newly expanded family requires relinquishing attachment to doing it all independently or perfectly. Allow loved ones to contribute through meals, errands help or just holding a baby while you nap. Receive this grace. Trust your inner guidance to set the pace, meet your needs gently, and write realistic expectations for this season overflowing with joy, change and profound self discovery.

<u>Setting Realistic Postpartum Nutrition Goals</u>
During pregnancy, your singular nutritional priority involves nourishing the rapidly developing baby through balanced macronutrients, vitamins, minerals and antioxidants. Yet the moment a baby makes their long-awaited debut, attention rightly fixates on that tiny new person wholly dependent on your care rather than self-focused goals. The postpartum period ushers in distinctly different nutritional aims centred around healing, restoring depleted reserves and adjusting to wildly fluctuating needs.

What should you realistically expect from your postpartum body still rebalancing after the marathon feat of labour, delivery and now milk production? How can you establish nutrition goals upholding your expanded family's wellbeing during this profound transition? Success stems from flexibly adapting to support changing needs with wisdom and patience instead of rigid expectations destined to fail.

Adapt to Your Appetite

During late pregnancy, rising levels of appetite-stimulating hormones like ghrelin and human placental lactogen drive increased hunger preparing your body for milk production. But fluctuating hormones, digestive changes and sheer fatigue often suppress appetite for the first couple postpartum weeks instead. Pressure to force feed generally backfires, undermining intuitive signals, so respect when your body naturally cycles between ravenous hunger and disinterest within a single day.

Rather than fixating on calories, protein grams or meal timing, allow appetite to guide when and what to eat with gentleness. Softer foods like soups, smoothies and bone broths often appeal most initially before gradually progressing back to heartier proteins, produce and complex carbs. Stay curious and adaptive to the cues signalling what nurtures best today while knowing periods of low and voracious hunger ebb and flow.

Support Milk Supply

If breastfeeding, sustaining ample milk production to meet baby's needs makes or breaks their growth and development. Yet stressful situations quickly suppress output by elevating cortisol. Postpartum vitamins containing galactagogues like fenugreek, blessed thistle and fennel seeds help some women, but reducing sources of anxiety and inflammation while emphasising skin-to-skin bonding and optimal nutrition offer the most efficacious supply boosters.

Focus first on consistent hydration and grazing smaller meals with priority proteins every 2-4 hours. Brewer's yeast, oats and leafy greens contain milk-enhancing compounds while coconut oil provides easily digested MCTs to fuel production. Customise food choices honouring current cravings intuitively guiding you toward balance. Trust your body knows exactly how - and when - to make milk even if volumes seem inadequate to you. Output meets true needs.

Stabilise Energy

Wild hormonal shifts the first couple postpartum months ripple into rollercoaster energy no new mom can effectively address by sheer willpower alone. The key rests in streamlining obligations, lowering other stressors and maximising restorative rest. Use food as the steadying force through balanced blood sugar regulation. Seek complex carbs from fibre-rich whole grains, starchy veggies and fruits paired with each meal's protein and healthy fats.

Identify your personal triggers plunging energy into the basement - perhaps skipping meals/snacks, consuming excess caffeine or sugar, chronic dehydration, poor sleep quality or depleted iron stores. Explore food journaling, stress reduction practices like meditation and streamlining help with baby care and household tasks using temporary assistance until patterns stabilise. This too shall pass!

Promote Gradual Weight Loss

Media and celebrity culture pressure new moms to instantly "bounce back" to pre-baby body composition yet the safe postpartum weight loss timeline aligns more with the 9 months it took you to gain pregnancy pounds. Losing too rapidly while breastfeeding signals tapping into depleted muscle mass for amino acid components of milk which backfires by cratering your metabolism. Gentleness serves you both better long term.

During the first six weeks, focus solely on healing and establishing breastfeeding until your care provider clears exercise again. Then begin gradual movement like walking, swimming or yoga avoiding high intensity workouts that spike cortisol and signal the body to retain fat stores in circulation for milk making. Emphasise plenty of proteins, vegetables, healthy fats and complex carbs first before tracking calories as you transition into your new normal.

Celebrate Non-Scale Victories

Remind yourself daily through affirmations, mirror work or journaling all your postpartum body performs wondrously right as pregnancy pounds slowly melt away. Making milk alone burns substantial fat stores! Notice positive changes like easing aches and pains, breasts naturally adjusting capacity to baby's increasing demand, brightening energy, less breast tenderness and strength returning for cradling your little one.

Celebrate positive gains like sleeping longer stretches at night as the baby settles, getting out to walk together in sunlight, having energy to make a healthy meal, enjoying your favourite pre-pregnancy foods again or wearing a once too-snug top now fitting comfortably. Give yourself permission to feel proud of all this body can do without fixating only the number on a scale. Loving patience is the most powerful goal.

The postpartum period deserves compassion not rigid expectations around food or fitness. Set yourself up for success by planning quick, balanced snacks and meals, emphasise ample sleep/rest, recruit helpful labour saving assistance, practice self-care basics first before tackling complex self improvement goals. Allow your body time and space for profound transformation unfolding on its own timeline. This too shall pass! Savour the precious journey.

<u>Creating a Supportive Environment</u>
The first weeks and months after welcoming your precious new baby hold such treasured joy. Yet simultaneously, new mothers face monumental physical and emotional adjustments to meet relentless demands nursing, changing diapers, soothing cries through the wee hours and somehow fueling their depleted body amidst sheer exhaustion. Creating an environment supportive of your

postpartum transition eases the intensity so you can embrace this poignant special time without burning out.

What constitutes a supportive landscape as you navigate healing from delivery, rollercoaster hormones, erratic sleep, pouring boundless love into your little one plus recovering energy stores to meet mounting needs? Begin by appreciating filling your own cup requires help, simplifying obligations and outsourcing chores so you can wholly cherish bonding unfettered by pressures pulling you too thin.

Ask for and Accept Support

New moms often feel inexplicable pressure to perfectly handle solo caring for a newborn, breastfeeding challenges, postpartum mood swings, major sleep deprivation all while keeping household duties like laundry, cooking and cleaning on track. Yet overwhelmingly trying to "do it all" without help courts breakdown from sheer exhaustion and stress fractures self-confidence when the load outweighs human capacity.

Push past the inner voice minimising your efforts or insisting accepting help somehow signals failure. Remind yourself frequently: you just performed an incredible feat growing and delivering new life! Now vulnerability requiring interdependence makes space for others to contribute care through providing meals, help with baby soothing, household tasks. Delegate, outsource and let non-essentials slide. Everyone involved will be graciously relieved.

Streamline Responsibilities

In the same way a newborn's cries can suddenly erase all sense of priorities beyond meeting their needs, the postpartum period begs for temporarily streamlining everything not related to recovery, rest and taking exquisite care of yourself plus the baby. Drive away unnecessary burdens and obligations so you don't split focus from what matters most right now.

Pare down self-maintenance like simplifying beauty routines, limiting decision fatigue with easy wardrobe grabs, stocking quick healthy snacks and staple meal ingredients that don't require daily thought. Say no whenever possible - now is not the season for overextending yourself. Protect space for treasured bonding by shedding non-essential doing. Make room for just being. Reprogram how your household functions.

Nourish Intentionally

Postpartum nutrition needs soar as your depleted body must simultaneously heal from delivery, adjust raging hormones, withstand sleep deprivation all while producing milk outpacing caloric and nutrient intake. Yet new moms often overlook self-care so foundational to enduring chaotic days vibrantly. Carve out time for nourishing yourself well by planning balanced meals & snacks and taking supplements to fill nutritional gaps.

Stock your kitchen with simple wholesome staples like eggs, yoghurt, nut butters, hummus, frozen fruits/veggies for smoothies. Meal prep freezer-friendly recipes when baby naps so you always have leftover soup, chilli or entrees easily reheated one-handed while you continue nourishing your little one. Simplify the process of getting enough nourishment even amidst unpredictable schedules.

Honour Signals From Your Body

Tuning into your authentic needs and attending to them with care allows instinctual wisdom to guide this profound transition amidst upended routines. Notice when exhaustion necessitates putting the baby down for a nap so you can rest too. Realising skipped meals or snacks drain energy reserves crucial for milk production and patience. Seek sunlight's nourishment, therapy in tears, solace in stillness when the world feels too overwhelming.

Your body will signal precisely what nurtures recovery if you grow skills listening below the static noise of external shoulds and obligations. Therapy, life coaching and meditation all help discern inner guidance toward what energises versus depletes so you can act accordingly. Say no to draining relationships. Seek activities enlivening your spirit. Prioritise whole food nourishment, movement bringing joy and sanctuary through rest, reflection or connection. Give yourself what your soul longs for.

Postpartum marks an intensely vulnerable passage through which gently caring for your needs amidst radical change lays the foundation for thriving. You must be well nourished to feed another! Supportive conditions serve your transition by simplifying overloaded plates, recruiting help and reminding yourself regularly that by receiving love through this temporary season, your precious new baby will organically learn to value interconnected communities too as they journey through life. This time too shall pass.

<u>Developing a Positive Mindset</u>

Alongside the joy, awe and fulfilment coursing through new mothers, the monumental transition into the disorienting world of parenting often simultaneously overwhelms even the most capable women unaccustomed to utter dependence. Endless feeding sessions stealing nightly sleep combined with racing worries never silenced for long. Recovering a body still stitching itself back together after delivering new life proceeds non-linearly. Patience Helplessness arises when best efforts at soothing a distressed baby prove futile.

The postpartum rollercoaster dips women to unknown depths unless conscious measures shore up emotional reserves weakened by chaotic hormones, identity shifts and sheer exhaustion. Intentionally cultivating positive perspectives and grace toward changing capabilities buoys women through unpredictable rapids. Creating space for your authentic experience without judgement allows deeper maturation into motherhood's complexity to unfold.

Reflect On Gratitude

When frazzled nerves short circuit perspective, reflect proactively through a gratitude journal on the tender joys before you. Thank your body for sustaining this new life still wholly dependent on your milk and care. Appreciate beloved friends and family eager to lend helping hands when the load exceeds your limits. Notice awe in your baby's angelic sleeping face that erases frustrating prior hours.

Write love letters to your little one as encouragement for someday when parenting horses and pressures weigh you down. Even just five minutes meditating on thankfulness for snuggles, noises, smells, smiles, warmth and the honour of guiding another soul counters negativity bias evolution ingrained. Intentionally redirect thoughts toward positivity.

Reframe Perceived Weakness

Society's messaging around perfect mothering establishes unrealistic standards destined to defeat any woman, especially in the postpartum phase. When your best efforts to calm a crying baby still escalate distress, when utter fatigue dulls patience, when you desperately crave alone time, these represent human needs not personal failings. Challenges passing too shall morph into strengths gained through surrendering control illusion.

Give yourself radical permission to feel, release emotion and progress through storms even if timelines appear delayed. Making space for needed rest, receiving help from loved ones or setting baby down when exhaustion threatens safe care all demonstrate responsiveness, not weakness. You must nourish yourself first to fill the baby's needs. Struggles serve growth. Progress through with self-compassion.

Rewrite Limiting Narratives

Self-critical stories echoing through a new mother's thoughts undermining confidence require replacing with intentional rewriting centred on self-care, priorities and unconditional love for this infant teacher. "My best is good enough for today." "I am present and receptive to guidance." I lovingly allow my needs and baby's needs equal importance."

When urgency overrides self-nourishment, shift inner dialogue with, "By resetting and restoring myself now, I am better able to provide the care my baby needs in this moment and beyond." Bond with other mothers to release guilt over imperfect journeys. Share in sorority remembering all parents have stumbled through storms blindly, been humbled by helplessness and discovered untapped wells meeting challenges.

Tune Into Body Wisdom
Tension accumulated through long days and nights caring for a newborn begs release

through movement, stillness and connection with instincts below mental static. Deep belly breaths activate the parasympathetic nervous system even for just one minute between diaper changes and nursing sessions. Enjoy sunlight or grounding bare feet on soil while babywearing. Squeeze stress balls. Dance together to favourite songs.

Tune into signals from your body guiding intuitive mothering wisdom moment to moment. Does hunger need addressing with another snack? Do tight shoulders necessitate a hot shower's comfort? Might fresh air enliven foggy fatigue? Listen then act accordingly. Each time tension looms, consciously relax muscles while visualising stress flowing out as grace enters.

Adopting proactive positive habits strengthens new mothers to skillfully ride unpredictable waves. Manifest patience, adaptability and compassion toward your personal journey right where you stand today, not some idealised destination.

Progress through struggles may not fit neat narratives but always enables growth. By loving the process, the challenges, the very present mundane moments, your ability to mother this child expands exponentially. You've got this!

Chapter 3: The Core Elements of a Postpartum Diet

The Core Elements of a One of the foundational pillars of postpartum nutrition is a sufficient intake of protein. During this phase, your body requires an increased amount of this essential macronutrient for tissue repair, muscle recovery, and overall healing. This is especially crucial for breastfeeding mothers as they need to replenish their bodies with the nutrients expended during the birthing process and support the development of their newborns.

Incorporating protein-rich foods into your diet is key. We explore various sources such as lean meats, poultry, fish, legumes, and dairy, highlighting their nutritional benefits. These foods not only provide the necessary amino acids for tissue repair but also play a vital role in sustaining your energy levels, a critical aspect of postpartum recovery.

Healthy Fats

The discussion then shifts to the importance of healthy fats, particularly omega-3 fatty acids. These fats are not only essential for your own well-being but also contribute to the healthy development of your baby's brain. Sources like fatty fish, avocados, and nuts are explored, emphasising their role in hormonal balance, immune system support, and the overall cognitive development of your newborn.

Understanding the distinction between healthy and unhealthy fats empowers you to make informed dietary choices that align with your postpartum goals. We provide practical tips on incorporating these fats into your meals in a balanced way, ensuring that you enjoy both the taste and health benefits.

Complex Carbohydrates

Next, we delve into the world of complex carbohydrates, which serve as a crucial source of sustained energy. Postpartum fatigue is a common concern, and the right carbohydrates can help combat this. Whole grains, fruits, and vegetables take centre stage as we explore their fibre content and their positive impact on digestive health.

By incorporating a variety of complex carbohydrates into your diet, you not only provide your body with the necessary energy but also support your digestive system, which may have undergone changes during pregnancy and childbirth.

Hydration for Postpartum Wellness

This section emphasises the often-overlooked aspect of hydration during the postpartum period. Adequate fluid intake is vital, particularly for breastfeeding mothers, as it supports milk production and helps prevent dehydration. We discuss the benefits of water, herbal teas, and hydrating foods, offering practical tips on maintaining proper hydration levels.

Recognizing the signs of dehydration and learning strategies to prevent it ensures that you stay energised and maintain optimal bodily functions during this critical time.

Key Takeaways:
- Protein, healthy fats, and complex carbohydrates are essential for postpartum recovery.
- A varied diet incorporating lean proteins, omega-3-rich foods, and complex carbs supports overall well-being.
- Hydration is a crucial yet often underestimated component of postpartum wellness.

Practical Application:
- Create balanced meals that include a mix of protein sources, healthy fats, and complex carbohydrates.
- Tailor your diet to your individual preferences a**and dietary needs.
- Implement strategies to stay adequately hydrated throughout the postpartum journey.

<u>Essential Nutrients for Recovery</u>
Protein-rich Foods

Proteins are the building blocks of life, and during the postpartum period, they play a pivotal role in recovery. The demands on your body are high, whether you've had a vaginal delivery or a caesarean section. Protein is essential for repairing tissues that may have been stretched or torn during childbirth and for rebuilding muscle strength.

Sources of Protein:
1. Lean Meats: Incorporating lean meats like chicken, turkey, and lean cuts of beef provides high-quality protein without excessive saturated fats.
2. Fish: Fatty fish such as salmon and trout not only offer protein but also provide omega-3 fatty acids, crucial for both your recovery and your baby's development.
3. Legumes: Beans, lentils, and chickpeas are excellent plant-based sources of protein, offering fibre and various vitamins and minerals.

4. Dairy: Milk, yoghurt, and cheese are rich in protein and also provide essential calcium for bone health.

Benefits of Protein:
1. Tissue Repair: Proteins contain amino acids, the building blocks for repairing tissues damaged during childbirth.
2. Muscle Recovery: Strengthening muscles, especially in the abdominal and pelvic regions, is essential for regaining core strength postpartum.
3. Energy Support: Protein helps sustain energy levels, combating the fatigue often experienced during the postpartum period.

Guidelines for Consumption:
1. Balanced Intake: Aim for a balanced distribution of protein throughout the day to support consistent energy levels.
2. Snacking Smart: Choose protein-rich snacks, such as Greek yoghurt with nuts or hummus with vegetables, to keep you fueled between meals.

3. Hydration: Ensure adequate water intake to support the efficient processing of proteins in your body.

Healthy Fats

While the term "fat" often carries a negative connotation, healthy fats are crucial for postpartum recovery. Omega-3 fatty acids, in particular, are essential for both your well-being and your baby's brain development.

Sources of Healthy Fats:
1. Fatty Fish: Salmon, mackerel, and sardines are rich in omega-3s, supporting brain health and reducing inflammation.
2. Avocados: Packed with monounsaturated fats, avocados are not only delicious but also contribute to hormone production.
3. Nuts and Seeds: Walnuts, flaxseeds, and chia seeds are excellent sources of omega-3s and provide additional nutrients like fibre and antioxidants.

Benefits of Healthy Fats:

1. Brain Health: Omega-3 fatty acids are crucial for your mental well-being and play a role in preventing postpartum mood disorders.

2. Hormonal Balance: Healthy fats support hormone production, aiding in the regulation of various bodily functions.

3. Inflammation Reduction: Omega-3s have anti-inflammatory properties, which can be beneficial in the postpartum recovery process.

Incorporating Healthy Fats:

1. Balanced Meals: Include a variety of sources of healthy fats in your meals, ensuring a well-rounded nutrient intake.

2. Meal Preparation: Cook with olive oil or avocado oil to add healthy fats to your dishes.

3. Snack Choices: Snack on a handful of nuts or enjoy slices of avocado on whole-grain toast for a nutrient-dense option.

Complex Carbohydrates

Complex carbohydrates are the body's primary source of energy, and after giving birth, maintaining steady energy levels is crucial for your well-being.

Sources of Complex Carbohydrates:
1. Whole Grains: Brown rice, quinoa, and whole wheat products offer a rich source of complex carbohydrates along with fibre and essential nutrients.
2. Fruits: Incorporating a variety of fruits such as berries, apples, and oranges provides natural sugars along with fibre.
3. Vegetables: Colourful vegetables, including leafy greens, carrots, and bell peppers, are nutrient-dense sources of complex carbohydrates.

Benefits of Complex Carbohydrates:
1. Sustained Energy: Unlike simple sugars, complex carbohydrates release energy slowly, preventing energy crashes.
2. Digestive Health: The fibre content in complex carbs supports a healthy digestive system, alleviating common postpartum digestive issues.

3. Nutrient Density: Whole grains and vegetables offer a plethora of vitamins and minerals, contributing to overall postpartum recovery.

Incorporating Complex Carbohydrates:
1. Balanced Plate: Aim for a well-balanced plate with a mix of lean protein, healthy fats, and complex carbohydrates.
2. Snack Options: Choose whole fruits or whole-grain crackers with hummus as satisfying and nutritious snacks.
3. Meal Variety: Explore different grains and vegetables to keep your meals interesting and nutrient-rich.

Key Takeaways:
- Protein is vital for tissue repair, muscle recovery, and sustained energy levels.
- Healthy fats, particularly omega-3 fatty acids, support brain health, hormonal balance, and inflammation reduction.
- Complex carbohydrates provide steady energy, support digestive health, and offer essential nutrients.

Practical Application:

- Plan meals that include a balance of protein, healthy fats, and complex carbohydrates.

- Choose a variety of protein sources to ensure a diverse nutrient intake.

- Experiment with recipes that incorporate healthy fats and explore different complex carbohydrate options to keep your meals interesting and nutritionally rich.

<u>Hydration for Postpartum Wellness</u>

Hydration is a fundamental aspect of postpartum wellness often underestimated in its significance. After childbirth, your body's hydration needs increase, particularly if you're breastfeeding. Adequate fluid intake plays a crucial role in supporting your overall well-being during this transformative period.

The Importance of Hydration:

1. Breastfeeding Demands: For breastfeeding mothers, staying well-hydrated is essential as breast milk production increases the

body's demand for fluids. Dehydration can affect milk supply and lead to fatigue.

2. Postpartum Recovery: Proper hydration aids in the recovery process, helping your body heal from the stress of childbirth. It supports tissue repair, reduces the risk of urinary tract infections, and ensures optimal functioning of bodily systems.

3. Energy Levels: Dehydration can contribute to feelings of fatigue, a common concern in the postpartum period. Maintaining adequate hydration supports sustained energy levels, crucial for meeting the demands of caring for a newborn.

Hydration Sources:

1. Water: Pure and simple, water is the best hydrating option. Aim for at least eight 8-ounce glasses per day, and more if you are breastfeeding or engaging in physical activity.

2. Herbal Teas: Non-caffeinated herbal teas, such as chamomile or peppermint, contribute to your fluid intake. They also offer soothing properties that can be beneficial for postpartum relaxation.

3. Hydrating Foods: Incorporate water-rich foods into your diet, such as fruits (watermelon, cucumber) and soups. These not only hydrate but also provide essential nutrients.

Signs of Dehydration:

It's crucial to be aware of signs indicating dehydration, especially during the postpartum period:

1. Dark Urine: Dark yellow urine may suggest dehydration. Aim for pale yellow or light straw-coloured urine as an indicator of proper hydration.

2. Thirst: Thirst is your body's way of signalling that it needs more fluids. Listen to your body and respond promptly.

3. Fatigue and Dizziness: Dehydration can lead to feelings of exhaustion and dizziness. If you experience these symptoms, it may be a sign to increase your fluid intake.

Strategies for Maintaining Hydration:

1. Set Reminders: In the busyness of caring for a newborn, it's easy to forget to drink water. Set alarms or reminders on your phone to prompt regular hydration.

2. Always Have Water Accessible: Keep a water bottle within reach, whether you're nursing, resting, or engaging in daily activities. Having water nearby encourages consistent sipping throughout the day.

3. Hydrate Before and After Feeding: If breastfeeding, make it a habit to drink a glass of water before and after each feeding session to replenish fluids.

4. Monitor Temperature: Hot weather or engaging in physical activity increases fluid

loss. Adjust your fluid intake accordingly to compensate for these factors.

5. Limit Caffeine and Sugary Drinks: While coffee and sugary beverages can contribute to overall fluid intake, they should be consumed in moderation. Water and herbal teas remain the primary sources of hydration.

Hydration and Breastfeeding:

1. Increased Needs: Breastfeeding mothers have higher fluid requirements. Aim for an additional 16 ounces (about 500 mL) of water per day compared to non-breastfeeding women.

2. Listen to Your Body: Thirst is a natural indicator of your body's need for fluids. Respond promptly to thirst cues to support both your hydration and milk production.

3. Monitor Baby's Diapers: Your baby's wet diapers are a good indicator of their hydration. If your baby is producing an

adequate number of wet diapers, it suggests they are receiving sufficient milk, which is directly influenced by your hydration status.

Key Takeaways:
- Hydration is crucial for postpartum wellness, supporting recovery, energy levels, and breastfeeding.
- Water, herbal teas, and hydrating foods are essential sources of fluids.
- Signs of dehydration include dark urine, thirst, fatigue, and dizziness.

Practical Application:
- Prioritise regular sips of water throughout the day, setting reminders if necessary.
- Keep water accessible in your breastfeeding area and around the house.
- Pay attention to signs of dehydration and adjust your fluid intake accordingly, especially during warm weather or physical activity.
- If breastfeeding, monitor your baby's wet diapers as an indirect indicator of your hydration and milk supply.

Chapter 4: Crafting Balanced Meals

Balanced meals are a cornerstone of postpartum nutrition, providing the essential nutrients your body needs for recovery, energy, and overall well-being. Crafting balanced meals involves a thoughtful combination of macronutrients (proteins, fats, and carbohydrates) and micronutrients to support your specific postpartum needs.

<u>Sample Meal Plans for New Moms</u>

Breakfast Ideas

- Option 1: Nutrient-packed Smoothie
    - Ingredients: Spinach, banana, Greek yoghourt, almond milk, and a scoop of protein powder.
    - Benefits: Provides a blend of protein, healthy fats, vitamins, and minerals. Ideal for a quick and nourishing start to the day.

- Option 2: Whole Grain Pancakes with Berries

- Ingredients: Whole grain pancake mix, topped with fresh berries and a dollop of Greek yoghurt.
- Benefits: Offers complex carbohydrates, fibre, antioxidants, and protein. A satisfying and delicious breakfast option.

Lunch and Dinner Recipes

- Option 1: Grilled Salmon with Quinoa and Roasted Vegetables
  - Components: Grilled salmon fillet, quinoa, and a variety of roasted vegetables (e.g., sweet potatoes, broccoli, and bell peppers).
  - Benefits: Rich in omega-3 fatty acids, complete proteins, complex carbohydrates, and a spectrum of vitamins and minerals.

- Option 2: Lentil and Vegetable Stir-Fry
  - Components: Lentils, stir-fried with a colourful assortment of vegetables (such as bell peppers, carrots, and snap peas), served over brown rice.
  - Benefits: Plant-based proteins, fibre, vitamins, and minerals. A hearty and vegetarian-friendly option.

Snack Options

- Option 1: Greek Yogurtparfait
  - Ingredients: Greek yoghourt, granola, and fresh berries.
  - Benefits: Combines protein, healthy fats, and antioxidants. A satisfying and convenient snack.

- Option 2: Hummus with Vegetable Sticks
  - Components: Hummus paired with sliced cucumber, carrot sticks, and cherry tomatoes.
  - Benefits: Provides plant-based protein, fibre, and a variety of vitamins. A nutritious and crunchy snack.

Mindful Eating Practices

Balanced meals are not just about the types of foods you consume but also how you approach eating. Mindful eating practices contribute to better digestion, satisfaction, and overall wellness.

Practical Tips:

1. Eat Mindfully: Sit down for meals without distractions, savouring each bite and paying attention to hunger and fullness cues.

2. Portion Control: Be mindful of portion sizes to prevent overeating. Listen to your body's signals of satiety.

3. Include a Variety of Colors: A colourful plate often indicates a diverse range of nutrients. Incorporate a variety of fruits and vegetables in different hues.

4. Hydrate: Drink water throughout your meals to aid digestion and maintain hydration.

5. Plan and Prep: Plan your meals in advance and engage in meal prep when possible. Having nutritious options readily available reduces the temptation of reaching for less healthy choices.

6. Enjoy Treats in Moderation: While focusing on nutritious meals, allow yourself occasional treats. Moderation is key to a sustainable and balanced approach to eating.

<u>Customizing Meal Plans for Individual Needs</u>
Recognizing that every postpartum journey is unique, customising meal plans based on individual needs and preferences is essential for long-term adherence to a healthy diet.

Customization Strategies:

Dietary Preferences: Tailor meal plans to accommodate dietary preferences, whether it be vegetarian, vegan, or specific cultural considerations.

Food Sensitivities: Identify and address any food sensitivities or allergies. Adjust meal plans accordingly to ensure optimal digestion and well-being.

Caloric Needs: Recognize that caloric needs can vary based on factors such as breastfeeding, physical activity levels, and individual metabolism. Adjust portion sizes and meal frequency accordingly.

Nutrient-Rich Ingredients: Prioritise nutrient-rich ingredients that align with your specific postpartum goals. For example, focus on foods rich in iron if you experienced significant blood loss during childbirth.

Gradual Changes: If making dietary changes, implement them gradually. This allows for a more sustainable adjustment and reduces the likelihood of feeling overwhelmed.

Key Takeaways:
- Crafting balanced meals involves a thoughtful combination of proteins, healthy fats, and complex carbohydrates.
- Sample meal ideas for breakfast, lunch, and dinner provide a variety of nutrients necessary for postpartum recovery.
- Mindful eating practices contribute to better digestion, satisfaction, and overall wellness.

Practical Application:

- Experiment with different meal combinations to find what works best for your taste preferences and dietary needs.

- Incorporate a variety of whole foods, including fruits, vegetables, lean proteins, and whole grains, to ensure a diverse nutrient intake.

- Practise mindful eating by being present during meals, paying attention to hunger and fullness cues, and enjoying the flavours of your food.

Chapter 5: Addressing Dietary Challenges

Among the many monumental transitions new parenthood brings, nourishing your body well often slides down the priority list behind caring for a needy newborn. Yet healing and revitalising your depleted reserves now lays the foundation for effectively meeting demands ranging from erratic sleeplessness to learning breastfeeding's rhythms. Ignoring nutrition threatens illness, slow recovery, infections, low energy and milk supply struggles.

But what if food brings more discomfort than nourishment in this tender phase? Navigating postpartum dietary challenges exacerbated by hormone fluctuations, a recovering digestive system, sheer exhaustion and limited time for meal prep trips up even the most diligent mothers. These practical tips help you overcome hurdles blocking adequate nourishment so essential for resilience.

Relieve Constipation Naturally

Many new moms battle postpartum constipation as pregnancy's elevated progesterone relaxes its hold, digestion slows after physical delivery stresses, pain meds cause backup and dehydration concentrates stool. Haemorrhoids worsen throbbing discomfort making elimination frightful. Nip bloating and hardness in the bud through diet improvements before reaching for laxatives.

Drink plenty of fluids like water, herbal teas and bone broths. Eat prunes or soaked chia seeds as natural stool softeners. Increase dietary fibre through whole grains, beans, veggies, nuts and seeds to bulk and moisten. Move daily, even just short gentle walks to stimulate motility. Probiotic foods like yoghurt and fermented pickles or supplements help rebalance gut flora thrown off by antibiotics. Consider magnesium supplements improving water retention in the colon for easier passages.

Soothe Heartburn & Reflux

Between digestion slowing thanks to residual progesterone, increased stomach pressure from a uterus shrinking back down and hormones relaxing the esophageal sphincter, many new mothers contend with postpartum heartburn, acid reflux or GERD. Spitting up milk compounds the problem with choking sensations and chest burning. Avoiding dietary triggers eases symptoms sans medications.

Skip aggravators like spicy foods, chocolate, caffeine, alcohol and large meals. Eat smaller portions more frequently instead of overfilling your stomach. Stay upright for at least an hour post-meals allowing gravity to keep gastric acid from splashing backwards. Calcium-rich foods help receptors closing off the oesophagus but avoid iron absorption. Acid reducers like almond milk, oatmeal, melon and ginger root naturally relieve discomfort.

Increase Appetite

Exhaustion from sleepless nights, digestive issues like nausea or constipation, pain from delivery recovery, overwhelming responsibility of newborn care...the postpartum period suppresses appetite for many women already depleted. Struggling to eat adequate calories and nutrients compromises milk supply and retard healing. Nourishing the body nourishing the baby requires consciously stoking hunger signals.

Dry toasted whole grain bread or crackers curb nausea better than heavy proteins until ready for heartier intake. Peppermint and ginger teas ease stomach upset. Tart cherry or pomegranate juice offer gentle nutrients. Meal prep freezer foods ready for quick eating without complex planning when energy nosedives. Recruit helpers so you can nap and restore appetite hormones like ghrelin. Small frequent portions of whatever appeals without pressuring quality over calories. This too shall pass!

Reduce Food Sensitivities

Thanks to intense hormonal shifts plus residual antibiotics and analgesics from delivery, new moms often react suddenly to previously well tolerated foods like dairy, gluten grains, shellfish, citrus fruits and nightshades. Always discuss significant changes with your provider to rule out mastitis and other infections. Meanwhile, tailor diet to ease upset.

Track reactions in a food journal to identify personal triggers then eliminate for 2-4 weeks before gradually reintroducing. Prioritise prebiotics like garlic, onions, asparagus and leeks feeding healthy gut flora hindering sensitivity reactions alongside daily probiotic foods. Choose gentle cooked vegetables and fruits over raw. Stick to familiar non-reactive proteins while healing. Peppermint, chamomile, marshmallow and ginger root herbs make soothing teas. Get checked for nutritional deficiencies exacerbating intestinal inflammation like zinc, omega-3s or magnesium. This too shall pass!

The postpartum diet deserves abundant compassion and adaptation to support healing with wisdom. Simplify nourishment by preparing balanced snacks and easy to digest meals ahead when possible. Hydrate extremely well and take a quality prenatal vitamin with iron until eating stabilises. Honour signals from your body above all, trusting innate cues toward what comforts versus inflames. Meet challenges gently, know they pass in time. This too shall heal!

<u>Coping with Food Sensitivities and Allergies</u>
Altered digestion ranks among the most frustrating for women seeking balanced nutrition to fuel recovery and breastfeeding. But gas, bloating and gastrointestinal discomfort often continue plaguing the postpartum period thanks to shifting hormones, prior antibiotics and anti-inflammatory meds slowing motility plus nerve inflammation from delivery stresses.

Suddenly formerly favourite foods trigger unpleasant reactions like abdominal pain, diarrhoea, headaches or skin flushing. You might suspect true food allergies especially if nursing a colicky or eczema prone baby. Both intolerances and bonafide allergies necessitate tailoring your diet to alleviate discomfort and identify triggering foods. Heal the gut for optimal wellness restoration.

Methodically Evaluate Reactions

Carefully log all foods and beverages consumed including ingredients and food sensitivities experienced like rash, gas, diarrhoea, abdominal cramps, stuffy nose or headache in a tracking app or notebook. Over 2-4 weeks patterns clearly emerge revealing your unique triggers. Note whether symptoms resolve by avoiding a food for a few days then reappear only when eating it again. Known common postpartum offenders include dairy, eggs, soy, wheat, shellfish, citrus and nightshades. Discuss significant changes with your provider to rule out infections.

Eliminate Aggravators Altogether

Once a food routinely provokes reactions, make the commitment to strict elimination without cheating for at least a month up to three. This requires vigilance reading all labels and asking questions when dining out but enables innate detoxification pathways to calm down. Reintroduced later in small quantities once stabilised. Some triggers like gluten grains in those with celiac disease may necessitate lifelong avoidance.

Support healing by emphasising antioxidant and prebiotic-rich real foods like colourful produce, garlic, onions, bone broth and gently cooked non-reactive proteins. Always prioritise allergen-free breast milk composition if the baby also shows food reactive symptoms like eczema, diarrhoea or congestion. Their developing immune system relies on your diet. The hidden gluten in soy sauce makes minute traces into your milk.

Strengthen Your Gut

All food intolerances and allergies relate closely to compromised intestinal permeability, frequently torn during pregnancy and postpartum thanks toHigh levels of inflammation, antimicrobials and hormonal shifts disrupt careful gates separating GI tract contents from immune surveillance. Undigested food particles then trigger reactions. Healing a leaky gut makes all the difference.

Reduce gut irritants by avoiding gluten, dairy, alcohol, NSAIDS like ibuprofen and excess sugar. Always check with your pharmacist and paediatrician about medications passing into breast milk too. Amp up prebiotics from garlic, onion, asparagus and leeks which nourish healthy gut flora. Prioritise probiotic foods like unsweetened yoghurt, kefir, kombucha, kimchi, miso, sauerkraut. Target 30-50 billion CFUs daily from high quality, third party verified probiotic supplements including saccharomyces and soil based species uniquely soothing intestinal tissues. L-glutamine amino acid also heals leaky gut excellently.

Substitute Nutritious Alternatives

Eliminating dietary allergens and sensitivities need not diminish flavour or nutrition. Substitute irritating cow's milk with coconut milk yoghurt and kefir, rich in gut healing Medium chain triglycerides(MCTs). Swap wheat for gentle oat, rice or nut-based gluten free grains still offering filling fibre and protein. Instead of inflammatory factory-farmed eggs, seek out pastured versions more digestible thanks to thick vitamin K2 rich yolks from hens eating a diverse diet. Organic produce avoids GMO and pesticide residues aggravating intestinal health.

Focus First on Anti-Inflammatory Foods

Ultimately reducing intestinal fire and Immune alarms necessitates basing intake around abundantly nutritious anti-inflammatory foods. Skipping trigger items gets you halfway there but proactively choosing colours from plants, particularly gently cooked vegetables, adds digestion-soothing fibre. Healthy fats like olive oil, avocado, nuts/seeds, fatty fish help resolve inflammation naturally and balance gut flora. Stay hydrated, emphasise easily absorbed bone broths and introduce new foods slowly once eliminating aggravators. This too shall heal!

<u>Handling Digestive Issues Postpartum</u>
Digestive issues can be a common concern for postpartum women, ranging from constipation to bloating and indigestion. Understanding and effectively managing these challenges is crucial for promoting overall well-being during the postpartum period.

<u>Understanding Digestive Issues Postpartum</u>

Common Digestive Issues:

Postpartum women may experience various digestive challenges, often stemming from hormonal fluctuations, changes in dietary habits, or the physical strain of childbirth. The most prevalent issues include:

1. Constipation: Reduced bowel movements can occur due to factors such as dehydration, changes in diet, or the lingering effects of medications used during childbirth.

2. Bloating: Hormonal changes and slowed digestion can contribute to bloating, causing discomfort and a feeling of fullness.

3. Indigestion: Changes in eating patterns, hormonal fluctuations, and stress may lead to indigestion, characterised by discomfort or pain in the upper abdomen.

Strategies for Managing Digestive Issues

Practical Tips:

1. Hydration is Key:

   - Adequate water intake is crucial for maintaining healthy digestion. Ensure you are drinking enough fluids throughout the day to prevent constipation.

2. Fibre-Rich Diet:

   - Include high-fibre foods such as whole grains, fruits, and vegetables in your diet. Fibre promotes regular bowel movements and alleviates constipation.

3. Regular Physical Activity:**

   - Gentle exercise, such as walking or postpartum-friendly yoga, can stimulate digestion and alleviate bloating.

4. Small, Frequent Meals:

   - Instead of large meals, opt for smaller, more frequent meals to ease the digestive process and minimise indigestion.

5. Probiotic Foods:

   - Incorporate probiotic-rich foods like yoghurt, kefir, or fermented vegetables to support the balance of gut bacteria and promote digestive health.

6. Avoid Trigger Foods:
   - Identify and avoid foods that may trigger digestive discomfort. Common culprits include spicy foods, caffeine, and gas-producing vegetables.

7. Mindful Eating:
   - Practise mindful eating by chewing food thoroughly and savouring each bite. This can aid digestion and prevent overeating.

<u>Seeking Professional Guidance</u>
Persistent or severe digestive issues may require consultation with healthcare professionals:

1. Healthcare Provider:
   - Discuss any persistent digestive concerns with your healthcare provider to rule out underlying medical issues.

2. Registered Dietitian:

- A registered dietitian can offer personalised dietary recommendations to address specific digestive challenges.

3. Pelvic Floor Physical Therapist:
    - For postpartum women, consulting with a pelvic floor physical therapist can be beneficial in addressing issues related to pelvic floor function, which may impact digestion.

Key Takeaways:
- Common digestive issues postpartum include constipation, bloating, and indigestion.
- Strategies for managing digestive issues include hydration, a fibre-rich diet, regular physical activity, and seeking professional guidance when needed.

Practical Application:
- Integrate fibre-rich foods, probiotics, and mindful eating practices into your daily meals.
- Stay hydrated by consuming an adequate amount of water throughout the day.

- Engage in gentle physical activity and consider professional consultation for persistent or severe digestive issues.

Balancing Dietary Restrictions with Nutritional Needs

For new moms navigating postpartum life, balancing dietary restrictions with essential nutritional needs is a delicate yet crucial task. Let's delve into practical strategies for maintaining a well-rounded and nourishing diet while accommodating any dietary restrictions that may arise.

Identifying Dietary Restrictions

Common Dietary Restrictions:

Postpartum women may encounter various dietary restrictions due to factors such as food sensitivities, allergies, cultural or ethical choices, or medical recommendations.

1. Food Sensitivities: Hormonal changes postpartum can heighten sensitivities to certain foods, leading to digestive discomfort or other symptoms.

2. Allergies: Pre-existing or newly developed allergies may necessitate the avoidance of specific foods to prevent adverse reactions.

3. Cultural or Ethical Choices: Some individuals may follow specific dietary practices based on cultural or ethical considerations, influencing food choices.

4. Medical Recommendations: Certain medical conditions or postpartum recovery requirements may warrant dietary modifications.

<u>Strategies for Balancing Dietary Restrictions</u>

Practical Tips:

1. Nutrient-Rich Alternatives:
    - Identify nutrient-rich alternatives to replace restricted foods. For example, if dairy is restricted, consider fortified plant-based milk for calcium.

2. Consult with a Dietitian:

- Seek guidance from a registered dietitian who can create a personalised meal plan considering your dietary restrictions while meeting nutritional requirements.

3. Label Reading:
   - Develop the habit of reading food labels to identify hidden allergens or ingredients that may conflict with dietary restrictions.

4. Meal Preparation and Planning:
   - Plan meals in advance, focusing on diverse, whole foods that align with your dietary restrictions and nutritional goals.

5. Supplementation if Necessary:
   - In consultation with healthcare professionals, consider supplements to address any potential nutrient gaps resulting from dietary restrictions.

6. Communication with Others:
   - Clearly communicate dietary restrictions to friends, family, or caregivers involved in meal preparation to ensure a supportive environment.

<u>Embracing Variety within Restrictions</u>

Practical Approaches:

1. Explore New Foods:
   - Embrace the opportunity to explore and incorporate new, nutrient-dense foods that align with dietary restrictions.

2. Experiment with Recipes:
   - Adapt favourite recipes to fit within dietary restrictions, using creative substitutions without compromising nutritional value.

3. Connect with Support Groups:
   - Engage with support groups or communities that share similar dietary restrictions for inspiration, advice, and recipe ideas.

4. Mindful Eating Practices:
   - Practise mindful eating to enhance the overall dining experience and promote

satisfaction within the constraints of dietary restrictions.

Key Takeaways:
- Identify and understand specific dietary restrictions, whether they stem from sensitivities, allergies, cultural choices, or medical recommendations.
- Utilise practical strategies, including nutrient-rich alternatives, consultation with a dietitian, label reading, and meal planning, to balance dietary restrictions with nutritional needs.
- Embrace variety within restrictions by exploring new foods, experimenting with recipes, connecting with support groups, and practising mindful eating.

Chapter 6: Fitness and Postpartum Nutrition

The postpartum period represents a unique and transformative time for women, and the integration of fitness and nutrition is paramount for overall well-being. This chapter will provide a detailed exploration of the importance of fitness, the role of nutrition, and practical guidelines for effectively combining the two during the postpartum journey.

<u>The Importance of Postpartum Fitness</u>

Physical and Emotional Benefits

Postpartum fitness is not just about shedding pregnancy weight; it plays a crucial role in physical and emotional recovery. Here are key benefits:

1. Muscle Recovery: Engaging in targeted exercises aids in the recovery of muscles strained during pregnancy and childbirth, promoting overall strength and functionality.

2. Mood Enhancement: Physical activity triggers the release of endorphins, contributing to improved mood and reduced feelings of postpartum depression and anxiety.

3. Increased Energy Levels: Despite the fatigue that often accompanies new motherhood, regular exercise can actually boost energy levels, assisting in the demands of caring for a newborn.

Restoring Core Strength and Stability

The core undergoes significant changes during pregnancy, and rebuilding its strength is crucial postpartum:

1. Pelvic Floor Exercises: Kegels and other pelvic floor exercises help restore strength and stability, addressing common issues like incontinence.

2. Abdominal Workouts: Gradual incorporation of safe abdominal exercises

assists in reactivating and strengthening the core muscles.

Gradual Progression

Postpartum fitness should be approached with patience and gradual progression:

1. Listen to Your Body: Pay attention to cues and avoid pushing too hard too soon. Each woman's postpartum journey is unique, and exercises should be tailored to individual comfort levels.

2. Professional Guidance: Consider consulting with a postpartum fitness specialist or physical therapist to ensure a safe and effective exercise routine.

<u>The Role of Postpartum Nutrition in Fitness</u>

Nutrient-Dense Diet for Recovery

Proper nutrition is the foundation for postpartum recovery and fitness success:

1. Protein for Repair: Adequate protein intake supports tissue repair and muscle recovery, especially crucial for women engaging in postpartum fitness routines.

2. Healthy Fats for Energy: Essential fatty acids contribute to sustained energy levels, crucial for both daily activities and workout sessions.

3. Carbohydrates for Endurance: Complex carbohydrates provide a steady source of energy, supporting endurance during workouts.

Hydration and Exercise Performance

Hydration is a critical element for both postpartum recovery and exercise performance:

1. Pre-Workout Hydration: Adequate water intake before exercise ensures optimal performance and reduces the risk of dehydration.

2. Post-Workout Replenishment: Rehydrate post-exercise to replace fluids lost through sweat and support recovery.

Practical Guidelines for Combining Fitness and Nutrition

Creating a Balanced Fitness Routine

1. Incorporate Variety: Include a mix of cardiovascular exercises, strength training, and flexibility work for a well-rounded routine.

2. Gradual Intensity: Begin with low-intensity exercises and gradually increase intensity as strength and stamina improve.

3. Postpartum-Friendly Workouts: Opt for workouts specifically designed for postpartum women, focusing on rebuilding the core and pelvic floor.

Meal Planning for Active Moms

1. Pre-Workout Nutrition: Consume a balanced meal or snack 1-2 hours before exercise, incorporating a mix of carbohydrates and protein for sustained energy.

2. Post-Workout Nutrition: Prioritise a post-exercise meal or snack within the first hour, emphasising protein for muscle repair and carbohydrates for replenishing glycogen stores.

3. Hydration Throughout the Day: Stay well-hydrated throughout the day, considering increased fluid needs during both postpartum recovery and exercise.

<u>Overcoming Challenges in Postpartum Fitness and Nutrition</u>

Time Constraints and Scheduling

1. Short, Intense Workouts: Opt for shorter, more intense workouts that can be integrated into busy schedules.

2. Schedule Prioritisation: Treat workouts as non-negotiable appointments, prioritising self-care for physical and mental well-being.

Balancing Nutritional Needs with Dietary Restrictions

1. Consult with Professionals: Seek guidance from a registered dietitian to create a personalised nutrition plan that accommodates any dietary restrictions.

2. Adaptation and Flexibility: Be adaptable in finding alternatives for restricted foods, exploring new recipes that align with nutritional needs.

<u>Celebrating Progress and Self-Care</u>

Acknowledging Achievements

1. Celebrate Small Wins: Recognize and celebrate every achievement, no matter how small, to stay motivated and positive.

2. Body Positivity: Embrace the changes in your body and focus on overall health and well-being rather than external appearances.

Self-Care Practices

1. Rest and Recovery: Prioritise sufficient rest and recovery days to allow the body to heal and rejuvenate.

2. Mindful Eating: Practise mindful eating, savouring each bite and fostering a positive relationship with food.

A Holistic Approach to Postpartum Well-Being

In summary, the journey of postpartum fitness and nutrition is a holistic one, intertwining physical activity with nourishment. By embracing gradual progress, prioritising a nutrient-dense diet, and overcoming challenges with adaptability, new moms can achieve a balanced and sustainable approach to postpartum well-being. The key lies in self-care, acknowledging achievements, and recognizing the interconnectedness of fitness and nutrition on the road to recovery and vitality.

Chapter 7: Nourishing Your Mental Well-being

The postpartum period is a transformative journey that extends beyond physical recovery. Nourishing your mental well-being is essential for overall health and happiness during this time. We will explore the multifaceted aspects of mental well-being, providing comprehensive insights and practical strategies for new moms.

The Importance of Mental Well-being in the Postpartum Period

Understanding Postpartum Mental Health
Postpartum mental health encompasses a spectrum of experiences, from the baby blues to more severe conditions like postpartum depression and anxiety. Recognizing the importance of mental well-being is the first step towards building a resilient and positive mindset.

1. The Baby Blues: Common in the first few weeks postpartum, the baby blues involve

mild mood swings, tearfulness, and feelings of vulnerability. These typically resolve on their own.

2. Postpartum Depression: A more persistent and severe form of mood disorder that affects daily functioning. It requires professional intervention and support.

3. Postpartum Anxiety: Characterised by excessive worry, fear, or panic attacks, postpartum anxiety can be overwhelming and impact a mother's ability to care for herself and her baby.

The Impact of Mental Well-being on Physical Health

1. Stress and Immune Function: Chronic stress can compromise the immune system, making the body more susceptible to illness. Prioritising mental well-being supports overall health.

2. Cognitive Function: A positive mental state enhances cognitive function, improving

decision-making, memory, and problem-solving skills.

3. Sleep Quality: Mental well-being directly influences sleep quality. Addressing mental health concerns contributes to better sleep hygiene.

Practical Strategies for Nurturing Mental Health

Building a Support System

1. Open Communication: Foster open communication with your partner, family, and friends about your emotions and challenges.

2. Professional Support: Seek the guidance of mental health professionals, such as therapists or counsellors, to navigate complex emotions.

3. Peer Support Groups: Engage with other new moms through support groups, sharing

experiences and advice to create a sense of community.

Self-Care Practices for Mental Well-being

1. Prioritise Personal Time: Set aside moments for self-care, even if brief, to recharge and focus on personal well-being.

2. Mindfulness and Meditation: Incorporate mindfulness techniques and meditation into your routine to promote mental clarity and stress reduction.

3. Creative Outlets: Explore creative activities such as journaling, art, or music to express emotions and foster a sense of accomplishment.

Healthy Lifestyle Habits

1. Balanced Nutrition: A well-balanced diet supports not only physical health but also mental well-being. Include nutrient-rich foods for optimal brain function.

2. Regular Exercise: Physical activity releases endorphins, promoting a positive mood. Incorporate gentle exercises like walking or postpartum yoga.

3. Adequate Sleep: Prioritise sleep hygiene to ensure sufficient and restful sleep, a cornerstone of mental health.

<u>Coping Strategies for Emotional Challenges</u>

Managing Stress

1. Identify Stressors: Recognize and address specific stressors, whether related to parenting, relationships, or personal expectations.

2. Stress-Reducing Techniques: Practise stress-reducing techniques such as deep breathing, progressive muscle relaxation, or guided imagery.

Overcoming Feelings of Isolation

1. Connection with Others: Actively seek social connections, even in small doses, to counter feelings of isolation.

2. Virtual Platforms: Utilise virtual platforms for communication, connecting with friends, family, or support groups.

Handling Mom Guilt

1. Redefine Expectations: Set realistic expectations for yourself, recognizing that perfection is unattainable.

2. Positive Affirmations: Incorporate positive affirmations into your daily routine to counteract negative thoughts and reinforce self-compassion.

Addressing Postpartum Depression and Anxiety

Recognizing Warning Signs

1. Persistent Sadness or Anxiety: Unrelenting feelings of sadness or anxiety beyond the

initial postpartum period may indicate a more serious concern.

2. Changes in Sleep and Appetite: Disruptions in sleep patterns or significant changes in appetite may be indicative of underlying mental health issues.

Seeking Professional Help

1. Consulting with a Healthcare Provider: Reach out to your healthcare provider if you experience persistent emotional challenges for a thorough assessment.

2. Therapeutic Interventions: Therapies such as cognitive-behavioural therapy (CBT) or medication may be recommended based on the severity of symptoms.

<u>Fostering a Positive Motherhood Mindset</u>

Embracing Imperfections

1. Acceptance of Reality: Embrace the imperfections of motherhood,

understanding that challenges are a natural part of the journey.

2. Celebrating Small Wins: Acknowledge and celebrate small victories, fostering a positive mindset amid the daily trials of parenthood.

Setting Realistic Expectations

1. Flexible Goal-Setting: Set realistic and flexible goals, allowing room for adjustments based on the unpredictability of parenthood.

2. Celebrating Personal Growth: Recognize the growth that comes with each challenge, viewing them as opportunities for personal development.

<u>Nurturing Mental Well-being Beyond the Postpartum Period</u>

Long-Term Strategies

1. Continued Self-Care: Establish self-care practices as an ongoing part of your routine, adapting them to your evolving needs.

2. Communication with Support System: Maintain open communication with your support system, seeking assistance when needed and sharing your emotional journey.

Evolution of Priorities

1. Adapting to Changes: Accept and adapt to the evolving demands of parenthood, recognizing that priorities and challenges will shift over time.

2. Professional Check-Ins: Periodically check in with mental health professionals for continued guidance and support.

Chapter 8: Diet Plan for Postpartum Moms

After the marathon of pregnancy culminates in childbirth, new mamas eager to reclaim their body and health often push overly hard through exercise and rigid dieting. But much deserved self-compassion better supports this tender transition through the first 6 weeks focused wholly on rest, bonding and full nourishment fueling recovery. Creating a personalised postpartum diet plan centred around simplified nutrition empowers healing.

Stock a Nourishing Pantry

Begin by taking inventory of your kitchen to identify any gaps needing restocking with broad spectrum whole food nourishment. Keep hunger, headaches and fatigue at bay through always having easy snacking staples readily available.

Good proteins to have on hand include: eggs, canned fish like salmon or sardines, Greek yoghurt, cottage cheese, nuts, nut butters, beans and lentils. Frozen fruits, leafy greens and vegetables offer quick smoothie prep or sides to meals. Stock up on healthy fats from olive oil, coconut oil, ghee, avocados. Choose complex carbohydrates like oats, amaranth, quinoa, squash, root vegetables.

Hydration forms a pillar for milk supply and recovery via coconut water, herbal teas, broths and water always available. Round out your healing pantry with fermented foods aiding digestion and gut health via kimchi, kefir, miso, pickles, and yoghurt.

Craft Nourishing Meals and Snacks

New mamasoften grab quick empty carb snacks enabling survival yet hunger again shortly thereafter. Stabilise intake through balanced meals and mini "meals" every 2-4 hours maintaining even energy and milk supply. Aim for lean protein, produce fruits and vegetables, healthy fats and slow burning carbs at each feeding.

Combinations might include: yoghourt with fruit, nuts and flax; omelette with spinach, avocado and berries; lentils with sweet potato and kale salad; peanut butter banana oat smoothie; bone broth soup with soft cooked veggies and quinoa; hummus and sliced peppers. Have snacks like hard boiled eggs, apples with nut butter, cheese slices with dry whole grain crackers ready to grab one-handed.

Simplifying Preparation
Take advantage of nap time moments to wash and prep fruits/veggies/greens for quick cooking or snacking throughout the week. Soups, stews and chilis freeze well for later reheating when energy nosedives. Stockpile lactation cookies, zucchini muffins, banana bread loaves to have nourishing snacks effortlessly on hand.

On chaotic days, smoothies allow throwing everything in the blender. Have supplies bedside for overnight feedings like protein bars, nut butter packets, coconut water and trail mix. Choose frozen produce to skip chopping when needed. Set up success through easily assembled nutrition.

Honour Your Authentic Needs

Every postpartum journey unfolds uniquely. Tune into your personal rhythms and preferences, indulging cravings in balanced moderation while respecting signals when favourite staples now trigger unpleasant reactions. Maybe meat seems unappealing but eggs, yoghurt and bone broth nourish. Perhaps salads distress your digestion but cooked greens or roasted veggies feel better. Attune yourself through journaling, meditation or counselling support if emotions complicate eating. This too shall pass! Sustain flexibility, curiosity and compassion.

<u>Weekly Meal Planners for Various Postpartum Stages</u>

The postpartum journey is dynamic, and nutritional needs evolve as new moms progress through different stages. This chapter provides detailed weekly meal planners tailored to address specific postpartum stages. From the early recovery period to the challenges of balancing motherhood, we'll explore nutritionally balanced meal options, snacks, and hydration strategies for each stage.

<u>Week 1-2: Initial Postpartum Recovery</u>

Key Nutritional Focus:

1. Hydration: Prioritise staying well-hydrated to support healing and milk production.

2. Nutrient-Dense Foods: Focus on easily digestible, nutrient-dense meals to aid recovery.

<u>Sample Meal Planner:</u>

Day 1:

- Breakfast: Whole grain toast with avocado and poached egg.

- Lunch: Chicken and vegetable soup with quinoa.

- Dinner: Baked salmon with sweet potato and steamed broccoli.

Day 2:

- Breakfast: Greek yoghourt with honey and a handful of almonds.

- Lunch: Lentil and vegetable stew.

- Dinner: Grilled chicken breast with quinoa and roasted Brussels sprouts.

Snacks:

- Fresh fruit slices.

- Hummus with cucumber sticks.

Hydration Tips:

- Aim for at least 8-10 glasses of water per day.

- Include herbal teas or infused water for variety.

Week 3-4: Establishing Routine and Increasing Activity

Key Nutritional Focus:

1. Protein Intake: Prioritise protein for muscle recovery, especially if engaging in gentle postpartum exercises.

2. Incorporate Iron-Rich Foods: Support iron levels, crucial for energy and overall well-being.

Sample Meal Planner:

Day 1:

- Breakfast: Spinach and feta omelette with whole grain toast.

- Lunch: Quinoa salad with grilled chicken, cherry tomatoes, and avocado.

- Dinner: Baked cod with lemon and herbs, served with brown rice and sautéed asparagus.

Day 2:

- Breakfast: Smoothie with berries, spinach, Greek yoghourt, and a scoop of protein powder.

- Lunch: Chickpea and vegetable stir-fry with brown rice.

- Dinner: Turkey meatballs with whole wheat spaghetti and marinara sauce.

Snacks:

- Trail mix with nuts and dried fruits.

- Cottage cheese with pineapple chunks.

Hydration Tips:

- Consume water-rich foods like watermelon and cucumber.

- Herbal teas with ginger for digestive support.

<u>Week 5-6: Gradual Return to Regular Activities</u>

Key Nutritional Focus:

1. Omega-3 Fatty Acids: Support brain health and mood with omega-3-rich foods.

2. Balanced Carbohydrates: Include complex carbohydrates for sustained energy.

<u>Sample Meal Planner:</u>

Day 1:

- Breakfast: Whole grain pancakes with fresh berries and a dollop of Greek yoghurt.

- Lunch: Quinoa and black bean bowl with grilled shrimp and avocado.

- Dinner: Grilled vegetable and salmon skewers with quinoa.

Day 2:

- Breakfast: Overnight oats with chia seeds, almond milk, and sliced banana.

- Lunch: Spinach and strawberry salad with grilled chicken.

- Dinner: Stir-fried tofu with broccoli and brown rice.

Snacks:

- Greek yoghourt with a drizzle of honey.

- Apple slices with almond butter.

Hydration Tips:

- Infuse water with citrus slices for added flavour.

- Green tea for antioxidants.

<u>Week 7-8: Full Engagement in Daily Activities</u>

Key Nutritional Focus:

1. Calcium-Rich Foods:** Support bone health, especially for breastfeeding moms.

2. Variety of Vegetables: Ensure a diverse range of nutrients from colourful vegetables.

<u>Sample Meal Planner:</u>

Day 1:

- Breakfast: Whole grain waffles with Greek yoghourt and mixed berries.

- Lunch: Quinoa and kale salad with grilled steak strips.

- Dinner: Baked chicken thighs with sweet potato wedges and roasted Brussels sprouts.

Day 2:

- Breakfast: Scrambled eggs with sautéed spinach and whole grain toast.

- Lunch: Mediterranean chickpea bowl with feta, cherry tomatoes, and olives.

- Dinner: Baked cod with mango salsa, served with quinoa.

Snacks:

- Cheese and whole grain crackers.

- Mixed fruit salad.

Hydration Tips:

- Include dairy or fortified plant-based milk for added calcium.

- Herbal iced tea with mint for a refreshing option.

Week 9-12: Embracing Full Postpartum Recovery

Key Nutritional Focus:

1. Incorporate Healthy Fats: Support hormone production and overall health.

2. Regular Intake of Fibre: Ensure optimal digestive health.

<u>Sample Meal Planner:</u>

Day 1:

- Breakfast: Smashed avocado on whole grain toast with smoked salmon.

- Lunch: Quinoa and vegetable stuffed bell peppers with a side of Greek salad.

- Dinner: Grilled shrimp and vegetable kebabs with quinoa.

Day 2:

- Breakfast: Acai bowl with granola, sliced banana, and a drizzle of honey.

- Lunch: Lentil and sweet potato curry with brown rice.

- Dinner: Baked chicken breasts with rosemary and garlic, served with roasted vegetables.

Snacks:

- Trail mix with dark chocolate and nuts.

- Cottage cheese with sliced peaches.

Hydration Tips:

- Coconut water for electrolyte balance.

- Infused water

with cucumber and mint.

<u>Post-12 Weeks: Sustaining a Balanced Postpartum Diet</u>

Key Nutritional Focus:

1. Maintain Adequate Hydration: Continue prioritising hydration for overall well-being.

2. Mindful Eating Practices: Pay attention to hunger and fullness cues for portion control.

Sample Meal Planner:

Day 1:

- Breakfast: Whole grain toast with almond butter and sliced strawberries.

- Lunch: Quinoa salad with mixed greens, grilled chicken, and a variety of colourful vegetables.

- Dinner: Baked salmon with a side of roasted sweet potatoes and green beans.

Day 2:

- Breakfast: Greek yoghourts parfait with granola, blueberries, and a sprinkle of chia seeds.

- Lunch: Chickpea and vegetable wrap with hummus in a whole grain tortilla.

- Dinner: Stir-fried tofu with broccoli, bell peppers, and quinoa.

<u>Snacks:</u>

- Fresh fruit slices with a handful of almonds.

- Rice cakes with avocado and cherry tomatoes.

Hydration Tips:

- Herbal teas with chamomile for relaxation.

- A daily glass of milk or fortified plant-based milk.

In conclusion, a flexible and adaptable approach to postpartum nutrition is essential, recognizing that every woman's journey is unique. These weekly meal planners provide a foundation for crafting a well-balanced diet throughout various postpartum stages. It's crucial to listen to your body, consult with healthcare professionals, and make adjustments based on individual needs and preferences. By nourishing the body with a variety of nutrients, new moms can support their recovery, energy levels, and overall well-being on the rewarding path of motherhood.

Chapter 9: Planning for Long-Term Health

The postpartum period marks the beginning of a transformative journey into motherhood, and planning for long-term health is a crucial aspect of this transition. In this chapter, we will explore the multifaceted elements of long-term health, including physical fitness, mental well-being, nutrition, and preventive care. This comprehensive guide aims to empower postpartum moms with knowledge and strategies to foster enduring well-being.

<u>Establishing Long-Term Health Goals</u>

Reflecting on Physical and Mental Well-being

1. Setting Realistic Goals: Begin by establishing achievable goals that align with your unique circumstances, considering both physical and mental aspects of well-being.

2. Prioritising Self-Care: Recognize the importance of self-care in sustaining long-term health. This includes regular exercise, mental health practices, and nurturing nutrition.

Incorporating Holistic Wellness Practices

1. Mind-Body Connection: Embrace practices that strengthen the mind-body connection, such as yoga, meditation, and mindfulness, for comprehensive well-being.

2. Balancing Priorities: Strive for balance in various life domains, including family, career, and personal pursuits, to enhance overall life satisfaction.

<u>Building Sustainable Fitness Routines</u>

Gradual Progression in Postpartum Exercise

1. Adapting to Changing Needs: Recognize that postpartum fitness requirements evolve. Begin with gentle exercises, gradually

increasing intensity and incorporating diverse activities.

2. Professional Guidance: Consult with a postpartum fitness specialist or physical therapist to ensure a safe and effective exercise routine that aligns with long-term fitness goals.

Diversifying Exercise Modalities

1. Cardiovascular Exercise: Engage in cardiovascular activities such as walking, jogging, swimming, or cycling to support heart health and maintain overall fitness.

2. Strength Training: Integrate strength training to build and maintain muscle mass, aiding in metabolism and providing functional strength for daily activities.

3. Flexibility and Balance: Include activities like yoga or Pilates to enhance flexibility and balance, contributing to injury prevention and overall well-being.

<u>Prioritising Mental Health for Longevity</u>

Consistent Mental Health Practices

1. Routine Check-Ins: Regularly assess your mental well-being, acknowledging emotions and addressing stressors promptly.

2. Therapeutic Interventions: Consider ongoing therapeutic interventions, such as counselling or support groups, to maintain mental health and build resilience.

Mindfulness in Daily Life

1. Incorporating Mindful Practices: Embed mindfulness into daily life through practices like mindful breathing, meditation, or mindful eating to foster mental clarity and emotional balance.

2. Stress Management Techniques: Develop a repertoire of stress management techniques, including deep breathing, progressive muscle relaxation, and positive visualisation, to cope with life's challenges.

Nurturing Long-Term Nutritional Habits

Continuation of Balanced Meal Planning

1. Diverse and Nutrient-Rich Diets: Sustain a diet rich in diverse nutrients, including lean proteins, whole grains, fruits, vegetables, and healthy fats, to support long-term health.

2. Mindful Eating Practices: Continue practising mindful eating, paying attention to hunger and fullness cues, and savouring the flavours of nourishing foods.

Adapting to Changing Nutritional Needs

1. Life Stage Adjustments: Recognize that nutritional needs may shift with different life stages, such as postpartum, breastfeeding, and beyond. Adjust your diet accordingly.

2. Consultation with a Dietitian: Seek guidance from a registered dietitian for personalised nutrition plans, especially during significant life transitions like

menopause or changes in dietary requirements.

Preventive Healthcare for Long-Term Well-Being

Regular Health Check-Ups

1. Annual Physical Examinations: Schedule regular check-ups with healthcare professionals for comprehensive physical assessments and screenings.

2. Routine Blood Tests: Monitor key health indicators, including cholesterol levels, blood pressure, and blood sugar, through routine blood tests.

Gynaecological Health

1. Regular Gynaecological Visits: Prioritise regular gynaecological visits for screenings, discussions about reproductive health, and addressing any concerns.

2. Contraceptive Consultations: If applicable, consult with healthcare providers about contraception options suitable for different life stages and family planning goals.

<u>Sustainable Habits for Postpartum Moms</u>

Sleep Hygiene for Longevity

1. Prioritise Quality Sleep: Establish and maintain healthy sleep patterns, ensuring sufficient and restful sleep for physical and mental well-being.

2. Consistent Sleep Routine: Implement a consistent sleep routine, including a calming bedtime ritual, to promote a restorative sleep environment.

Stress Reduction Strategies

1. Holistic Approaches: Explore holistic stress reduction strategies such as acupuncture, massage therapy, or engaging in hobbies to enhance overall well-being.

2. Time Management: Implement effective time management strategies to reduce stress associated with balancing various responsibilities.

<u>Embracing Changes and Celebrating Milestones</u>

Adapting to Life Transitions

1. Flexibility in Goals: Embrace the flexibility to adapt long-term health goals to accommodate life transitions, such as career changes, family growth, or personal pursuits.

2. Resilience in the Face of Challenges: Cultivate resilience to navigate challenges, understanding that setbacks are a natural part of any health journey.

Celebrating Personal Growth

1. Reflection on Achievements: Regularly reflect on personal growth and health achievements, celebrating progress and recognizing the journey.

2. Positive Self-Image: Foster a positive self-image

Conclusion

As we come to the close of this insightful journey through the pages of "Postpartum Diet Book for New Moms," we find ourselves at the threshold of a remarkable chapter in the lives of new moms. The adventure of motherhood is an ever-evolving odyssey, marked by the joys, challenges, and the relentless pursuit of well-being.

In these pages, we've delved deep into the core elements of postpartum health, unravelled the nuances of nutrition, celebrated the triumphs of balanced meal planning, and charted a course for long-term well-being. Our aim has been to empower new moms with the knowledge, tools, and inspiration to navigate the postpartum landscape with confidence, resilience, and a deep understanding of their unique needs.

The journey of postpartum wellness is not a linear path but a mosaic of experiences, each contributing to the masterpiece that is motherhood. From the early days of recovery to the establishment of balanced routines, and onwards to the sustained well-being that spans a lifetime, this guide has endeavoured to be a trusted companion, offering guidance, encouragement, and a touch of inspiration.

As we bid adieu to these pages, let us carry forward the essence of what we've explored. Let us remember the importance of self-care, the vitality of balanced nutrition, and the resilience embedded in the core of every new mom. May the wisdom shared in these chapters serve as a beacon of light during moments of uncertainty and a source of strength as new challenges and triumphs unfold.

To every new mom embarking on this extraordinary journey, know that you are not alone. Your path may be unique, but the collective spirit of motherhood weaves a tapestry of shared experiences and shared wisdom. Embrace the changes, celebrate the victories, and, above all, honour the incredible strength that resides within you.

As the pages of this book turn, may they symbolise the turning of chapters in your own story—each page a testament to growth, resilience, and the enduring beauty of the journey you've embarked upon. Here's to the countless moments of joy, the lessons learned in the face of challenges, and the unwavering spirit that defines the heart of motherhood.

In closing, let this be a reminder: You are strong. You are resilient. You are a beacon of love and nurturing. May your postpartum journey continue to unfold with grace, and may you find profound joy in the unfolding chapters of the extraordinary narrative that is your life as a new mom.

Wishing you boundless love, health, and an abundance of beautiful moments on this timeless journey.